Water Exercises
for Parkinson's

Maintaining Balance,
Strength,
Endurance,
and Flexibility

Ann A. Rosenstein

Foreword by Len Kalakian, Ph. D.

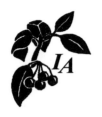

Idyll Arbor, Inc.

PO Box 720, Ravensdale, WA 98051 (425) 432-3231

Idyll Arbor, Inc. Editor: Thomas M. Blaschko

Photographs: Leroy Cech

2nd Printing, December 2003

Library of Congress Cataloging-in-Publication Data

Rosenstein, Ann, 1958-
    Water exercises for Parkinson's : maintaining balance, strength, endurance, and flexibility / Ann Rosenstein; forward by Len Kalakian.
        p. cm.
    Includes bibliographical references and index.
    ISBN 1-882883-49-7 (alk. paper)
      1. Parkinson's disease--Exercise therapy. 2. Aquatic exercises. 3. Parkinson's disease--Patients--Rehabilitation. 1. Title.

    RC382.R674 2002
    616.8'33062--dc21

                          2001051720

ISBN 1-882883-49-7

DEDICATION

To Tom Mraz

and all those who struggle with Parkinson's disease,
their partners, and their caregivers.

ACKNOWLEDGMENTS

This book could not have been written without the help of many talented and patient people. A special thank you to Tom Mraz and Vickie Lynn. Both have Parkinson's disease and graciously allowed me to use them as models for the exercises. Their dedication and hard work are an inspiration. Thank you to Ed Mako who acted as the companion to Tom and encouraged me to write this book. Thank you to Leroy Cech who did a wonderful job with the photography. Thank you to Osmund A. Wisness who also posed for some of the pictures. Thank you to Dr. Len Kalakian who did a masterful job of the first editing of the sections on Stretching and Exercises. Thank you to the management teams of the Burnsville YMCA, Burnsville Northwest Athletic Club, and The Marsh Club in Minnetonka, MN for allowing me to use their facilities during photo sessions. Thank you to Tom Blaschko for his excellent job of editing the entire book.

Last, but not least, a very special thank you to my husband Leo who helped with editing, pictures, cropping, and computer glitches. He also showed unwavering faith and encouragement, gave me love, strength, and support when I needed it most and never doubted my abilities.

Contents

Foreword

Ann Rosenstein has written a book on water exercise specifically for people who have Parkinson's disease and those associated with their care. Her book gives a good overview of the causes, treatments, and advances being made with regard to Parkinson's disease. She has thoroughly researched these areas and how they relate to water exercise. She discusses how exercising in the water is unique, since it helps a person maintain balance and supports a person's weight while protecting joints from injury. Water offers constant but gentle resistance for the muscles. Ms. Rosenstein has also included a section on water and pool safety. Being able to safely access a pool is just as important as knowing how to exercise in the water. Knowing what medications are available and how they affect a person is also important. Exercising when one is at one's best is always desirable.

When one acquires a label, such as Parkinson's, that label often conjures up preconceived notions about what the person with the label cannot do. When the label happens to be some disability, "dis" in the word dis-ability often overshadows ability. Disability labels, far from celebrating what is right, usually exaggerate what is wrong. Exaggerating negatives needlessly breeds under-expectations for persons upon whom labels have been conferred. Unfortunately, it is all too easy to become the sum product of "under-expectations" — our own and those from people around us.

Ms. Rosenstein's book is a label challenger. It is a book for people, those who happen to have Parkinson's but choose to live well. It is a book for people wishing to put individuality before labels. In this book, the reader will find detailed pictures of water exercises being portrayed with people who have Parkinson's disease. With the help of photos, the exercises are described in detail as to what they are and how they specifically benefit people with Parkinson's. Medical and fitness professionals know that exercise helps people with Parkinson's to maintain muscle strength and flexibility. This, in turn, helps the person retain independence for as long as possible.

While her message is directed toward people with Parkinson's, it bears broad efficacy for all people striving to approach life holistically. Holistic living is about mind-body unity, and belief in its merits date at least as far back as the ancient Greek philosopher Plato. Plato taught that a body functions best when supported by a well mind, and a mind functions best when supported by a well body. The term "well" should not be misconstrued; one becomes well when one achieves her/his unique potential. By example, one can be perceived as Mr. or Mrs. Universe, yet, for a variety of reasons, not be well, while someone else living life's final days in a hospice can be extraordinarily well.

Achieving wellness can be a tricky business, because sometimes we allow ourselves to become seduced by idealized pictures of life, extremes if you will. Often we measure ourselves against these ideals and extremes. When we do, typically we come away feeling unfulfilled, sometimes even demoralized. This need not happen, should not happen, and, for individual wellness, must not happen. Rightly, your responsibility to you is to be the best "you" that you can be. To accomplish this, according to Socrates (Plato's teacher), one must first "Know thyself," and then "To thine own self be true." This book is about knowing and being true to oneself, and particularly about being true to one's body in the mind-body equation.

Like Socrates (and my intent is not to exaggerate), Ms. Rosenstein is saying from the perspective of a holistic personal trainer, "Know thyself" and "To thine own self be true." Her book is a "How to" manual for people who wish to be all they can be. Within these pages, she and her clients celebrate the difference, indeed, the chasm, between being average and being normal. Being average with regard to any ability is really about not doing very much. Normal is about making and acting on the decision to become all one is really meant to be. Often, we tend to confuse average with normal, only because we see so much average around us. Ms. Rosenstein's book is a guide for bridging the fitness gap for persons with Parkinson's between average and normal. I believe the real message of Ms. Rosenstein's book is, "Why would I want to be average when I can be normal?"

Ms. Rosenstein's activities are tried and true. Her book is the only book I know of that specifically describes water exercises for people with Parkinson's disease. She discusses a unique approach about becoming an exercise partner for a person who has Parkinson's disease. Her clients, who have Parkinson's, also her models for this text, demonstrate how to cross the bridge that separates average from normal. This book is thoroughly researched and offers promise to those with Parkinson's disease. The bridge is waiting. The map is in your hands. Use it in good health!

Len Kalakian, Ph. D., Professor Emeritus
Adapted Physical Education
Department of Human Performance
Minnesota State University — Mankato

Introduction

People who have recently been diagnosed with Parkinson's disease and people who have been dealing with the disease for an extended period of time want to preserve their independent lifestyle. In order for their independence to be preserved, people with Parkinson's need to retain the physical functions of their bodies for as long as possible, especially flexibility, strength, and functional mobility. An exercise program is essential to achieve these goals. Such an exercise program is explained in great detail in this book, *Water Exercises for Parkinson's.*

This book is written for people who have Parkinson's disease, their families, and professional caregivers such as physical therapists, personal trainers, fitness instructors, nurses, and physicians. The book will help guide people with Parkinson's through a water exercise program as part of the overall management of their disease. Exercise will not cure or stop the progression of Parkinson's disease. Exercise, especially water exercise, will help to improve body strength and balance so the person is less incapacitated and able to lead an independent, active life for a longer period of time. Exercise improves balance and gait problems in people with Parkinson's, and improves their emotional well being by giving them a feeling of accomplishment.

Even though the exercises are to be performed by the person who has Parkinson's disease, those who are associated with the care of the person with Parkinson's need to review the material in this book with him/her. Sometimes people who have Parkinson's have a difficult time remembering tasks from one day to the next.

People with Parkinson's also do better when they learn to master one task at a time. This is where the caregiver, companion, spouse, or fitness trainer can be of help by reading through this book with the person with Parkinson's and by assisting him/her to master the exercises at his/her own pace.

Water Exercises for Parkinson's will present the importance of exercise as part of the overall treatment plan for people who have Parkinson's disease. The benefits of water exercises will be emphasized along with descriptions of helpful water exercises, workout programs, and safety during those exercises and workouts.

Basics of Parkinson's Disease

Parkinson's disease is not contagious or fatal, but it is chronic and progressive; its symptoms worsen over time. Parkinson's disease is a neurodegenerative condition that affects over one million people in the United States, with 50,000 new cases being diagnosed each year. Parkinson's disease affects one out of every 100 people sixty years and older. As people age, the chances of getting Parkinson's increases. In people 70 years and older, 1.5% to 2.5% have Parkinson's. Parkinson's disease also affects people younger than sixty. As many as 15% of people diagnosed with Parkinson's are fifty and younger. Because of the special needs of people with Parkinson's, the disease costs $20 billion a year.

The disease is named after Dr. James Parkinson, a London physician who described the syndrome in 1817 in a treatise titled *On the Shaking Palsy*. Parkinson's disease has plagued mankind for thousands of years. Egyptian hieroglyphs 4000 years old show depictions of people with Parkinson's disease symptoms. Symptoms of Parkinson's are also mentioned in ancient Greek and Roman writing. There are also descriptions of Parkinson's symptoms mentioned in the Bible.

Most people suffer from idiopathic Parkinson's disease (IPD). Idiopathic means "without known cause." IPD tends to affect one side of a person's body more than the other.

The four major symptoms of Parkinson's disease are rigidity, resting tremors, slowness in starting movement, and the loss of postural reflexes. Rigidity is the stiffness felt when trying to move the arms, legs, and neck. Rather than being able to move with a fluid motion, the person with Parkinson's feels stiff and has trouble bending at the joints. In unaffected people, muscles work in pairs such as quadriceps/hamstrings or biceps/triceps. Rigidity occurs when only one part of the muscle pair becomes strong, thus pulling the limbs and joints out of balance. Examples are continuously flexed elbows, curled toes, and stooped posture (also known as kyphosis). Resting tremors are involuntary tremors that are most pronounced when the body is at rest.

Slowness in starting a movement is called bradykinesia. Bradykinesia is the primary cause of the shuffling gait, small tight handwriting called micrographia, and expressionless facial patterns called Parkinson's facies. Bradykinesia is also defined as poverty of motion. The slowness of movement occurs when the brain must find an alternate path for neurological signals. Poverty of motion refers to the loss of normal animation in the muscles that continually change the position of the body and the face. People with Parkinson's may be attentive and alert inside but they will appear motionless until an outside stimulus causes them to move. Such stimuli can be clapping the hands or snapping the fingers. Bradykinesia is a major contributor to a shuffling gait. The legs are already stiff and heavy from rigidity. Combined with the slow movement and poverty of motion, a person with Parkinson's can only lift his/her leg for a short time before the muscles become fatigued. The same principle applies to micrographia and Parkinson's facies.

The combination of all four symptoms forces the person with Parkinson's into a stooped, unbalanced, and unsteady posture making physical movement, especially walking, difficult.

Secondary symptoms of Parkinson's disease include depression; emotional changes; memory loss; sleep problems; digestive problems; problems with chewing, swallowing, and speaking; and low blood pressure upon standing (postural hypotension). People with Parkinson's usually experience only some of these symptoms. For some people, Parkinson's disease may affect one side of the body more than the other. Some people may live with Parkinson's for many years before the symptoms become a real problem. It is not unusual for the disease to progress slowly over a 20 to 30 year period. However, without treatment, pronounced disability can occur in nine years or less. While we don't have a cure for Parkinson's yet, symptomatic medications, diet, and exercise help slow the disease's progress so people live with Parkinson's better and longer and are more able to maintain mobility and function.

The physiological changes associated with Parkinson's disease occur in the area of the brain called the substantia nigra. See Figure 1. As the disease progresses, 70%-80% of the neurons using dopamine as a signaling agent deteriorate. The basal ganglia, which connect with the substantia nigra, are a major center for the body's initiation and coordination of motor movements. Dopamine is an important neurotransmitter that is found in the brain and is vital to the normal functioning of the central nervous system. Dr.

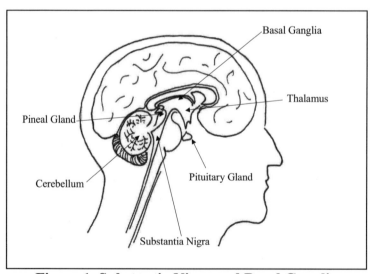

Figure 1. Substantia Nigra and Basal Ganglia

Arold Carlson from Sweden discovered the importance of dopamine, which acts as a chemical messenger between the brain cells in the basal ganglia.

When dopamine transmitters first begin to deteriorate and die, the person often experiences a set of vague complaints including restlessness, inability to sleep, and anxiety. Further deterioration leads to muscle rigidity and tremors. With the depletion of dopamine, balance and coordination are diminished. As a result, falling occurs more frequently. This is often the symptom that leads people to seek medical attention. As the disease progresses, falling increases, along with decreased mobility. This is why Parkinson's is sometimes referred to as the Falling Sickness.

Later in the progression of Parkinson's disease cognitive degeneration and dementia may be seen. Cognitive degeneration is characterized by memory loss, personality changes, and increased emotional imbalance. Family members, care givers and friends may notice the person with Parkinson's having trouble recalling recent events and becoming increasingly confused about days, dates, and familiar surroundings. Personality changes include increased passivity or increased aggressiveness, a lack of interest in hobbies, family, and socializing.

Profound memory loss and confusion tend to occur in the later stages of Parkinson's disease. About 14% to 20% of people in the more advanced stages of Parkinson's have cognitive dysfunction that is severe enough to interfere with daily living. Some experts indicate the percentage may be as high as 50%. When cognitive dysfunction is that severe, it is referred to as dementia.

Dementia is defined as a loss of intellectual abilities that are severe enough to interfere with occupational and social functioning. Dementia in Parkinson's disease is called subcortical dementia, which involves mood alterations, cognitive dysfunction, memory difficulties, and psychomotor retardation (bradyphrenia). Care givers will notice the slowing of movement or muscular activity associated with failing mental processes. People with Parkinson's disease who have bradyphrenia take a longer time to process instructions, information, and perform physical tasks.

Multiple methods of cueing may be required to help the patient figure out how to perform tasks such as the exercises in this book.

Subcortical dementia is thought to occur due to abnormalities in the multiple neurotransmitter systems found in the deep gray matter structures of the brain. The specific neurotransmitter systems affected are acetylcholine, norepinephrine, serotonin, dopamine, and somatostatin.

There is no particular cause for Parkinson's disease (PD). In the 1980's, it was thought that genetics played a part in whether or not a person got PD. It seemed that genetics played a role because 10% to 15% of PD cases had relatives who also had PD. Studies were done on twins, both identical and fraternal. It was found that when one identical twin had PD, the other had the same chance of getting PD as a non-identical twin. Therefore, Parkinson's disease seemed less likely to have a genetic cause.

A study published in the January 1998 issue of *The Journal of the American Medical Association* reported on 19,842 white male twins who had enrolled in the National Academy of Sciences/National Research Council World War II Veteran Twins Registry for suspected Parkinson's disease. The theory that genetics played a role in Parkinson's was tested and the researchers found that Parkinson's disease did not show up in both twins as was thought. Again, Parkinson's disease seemed to not have a genetic component.

Dr. Erin Montgomery, Jr. of the Cleveland Clinic Foundation conducted one study that sought to establish a genetic risk for Parkinson's. Dr. Montgomery was trying to establish if specific tests could identify the disease in children and siblings of patients with Parkinson's disease. The children and siblings of people with Parkinson's showed no apparent signs of the disease but were more impaired than normal people in the same age group.

Dr. Montgomery tested 80 first-degree relatives of Parkinson's patients against 100 control individuals by giving each group tests that calculated the degree of motor function, sense of smell, and emotional state. He found that 22.5% of the relatives of the people with Parkinson's scored in the abnormal range as opposed to 9% of the people in the control group. Among the children of people with Parkinson's, those who tested abnormal came from families where the parent with the disease was the father. This study suggested a possible genetic connection although environment is now considered a more likely factor.

Other researchers looked at the environment and discovered that neurotoxins, such as those found in pesticides, destroy the substantia nigra and can produce neurochemical changes like those found in PD. At the Stanford University's School of Medicine in California a study looked at the pesticide exposure of 496 people with Parkinson's and 541 disease-free people. The study found that those with Parkinson's disease were more than twice as likely to have been exposed in the past to insecticides in the home.

In Milan, Italy, at the Parkinson's Institute, researchers conducted a study comparing exposure to organic solvents and industrial hydrocarbon compounds and the risk of acquiring Parkinson's disease. Common compounds are benzene and toluene. The study involved 900 patients with Parkinson's disease. The study showed that of the 900 patients involved, those who were exposed to organic solvents and hydrocarbons developed symptoms of PD three years earlier than other patients with PD. Furthermore, the severity of their symptoms were proportional to the amount of hydrocarbons they were exposed to. Three types of industries were found to contribute 91% of the exposure. They are the petroleum, plastic, and rubber industries.

Just recently, Dr. Timothy Greenamyre and his colleagues at Emory University in Alabama discovered that the organic pesticide rotenone causes or contributes to Parkinson's disease in rats. In his study, rats were given low, steady doses of rotenone into their bloodstream over a period of one to five weeks. After the rats were exposed to the rotenone, they became stiff, slow moving, had tremors, and became hunched over. Dr. Greenamyre discovered that the pesticide destroyed the same brain cells that are destroyed by Parkinson's disease.

A more recent study was conducted by Deborah Cory-Slechta, PhD, University of Rochester School of Medicine and Dentistry and published in the December 15, 2000 issue of the *Journal of Neuroscience*. Dr. Cory-Slechta's team studied the effects two agricultural pesticides had on mice. The two chemicals studied were paraquat, an herbicide, and maneb, a fungicide. Farmers working millions of acres of farmland use these two chemicals. Paraquat is used on fruits, vegetables, corn, soybeans, and cotton to stop the growth of weeds. Maneb is used on tomatoes, potatoes, lettuce, and corn to stop fungi.

In the experiment, mice were exposed to each of the chemicals separately. After the exposure, the mice showed no signs of Parkinson's type symptoms. However, when the mice were exposed to both chemicals, they exhibited Parkinson's type traits that exactly matched traits found in people with Parkinson's disease. The mice that were exposed to the combination of paraquat and maneb had 15% fewer dopamine neurons and produced 15% less dopamine than the control mice.

Farmers often use both chemicals on the same crops in the same fields. First the farmer kills the weeds with paraquat and then goes back over the same crops with maneb, thus being exposed to the chemicals in tandem. It is not known how much exposure poses a risk or how much time elapses between the use of each chemical. Often paraquat and maneb are used at different times of the growing season. It is also unclear as to how much of the pesticides remain on the foods once they reach the consumer and if it is enough to cause concern. Maneb can leave a slight residue and paraquat leaves trace amounts. If both chemicals are on the food purchased by consumers, then they become exposed to the combination.

The study also indicated that older mice were more sensitive to the exposure of the combined chemicals. Cory-Slechta's researchers also found that mice that had the same genetic abnormality that causes some people to get Parkinson's were more vulnerable to the chemical combination.

In our environment, there are many combinations of pesticides, fungicides, herbicides, and other organic chemicals. This study indicates that combinations of such chemicals may contribute to the cause of Parkinson's disease even when the individual chemicals are thought to be safe. The most concentrated cases of PD are found among farmers in rural areas mostly in the Midwest, California, Florida, and the Northeast. People who drink well water are also at a greater risk of developing the disease.

The environmental connection between PD and pesticides is reflected in the chart put out by the National Parkinson Foundation. Dr. Abraham N. Lieberman, the Medical Director of the National Parkinson Foundation, wants to establish a Parkinson's Registry in order to have a more accurate account of who has PD and where they live. See the chart on the next two pages.

In order to get an account of who has PD, the sale of the Parkinson's drug Sinemet was tracked in each city, county, state, and zip code. The data shows that five states in the Midwest have the highest number of people with PD. They are also farming states where there is a high use of insecticides, herbicides, and fungicides.

The state with the highest concentration of PD cases is North Dakota followed by South Dakota, Iowa, Nebraska, and Minnesota. These five states also have populations whose ancestors are from Northern Europe (Germany, Norway, Sweden, and Denmark). This suggests a possible genetic predisposition towards PD.

Another case for environmental influence is from the tropics. For decades, atypical Parkinson's disease has affected people who reside in the tropics. Atypical Parkinson's or ATP differs from idiopathic Parkinson's in that atypical Parkinson's affects both sides of the body equally and ATP sufferers do not respond well to levodopa drug treatment. One such atypical Parkinson's is called Guam syndrome and affects the people of Guam. Those who have this form of Parkinson's have all of the classic symptoms such as tremors, muscle rigidity, slowness of movement, and poor balance.

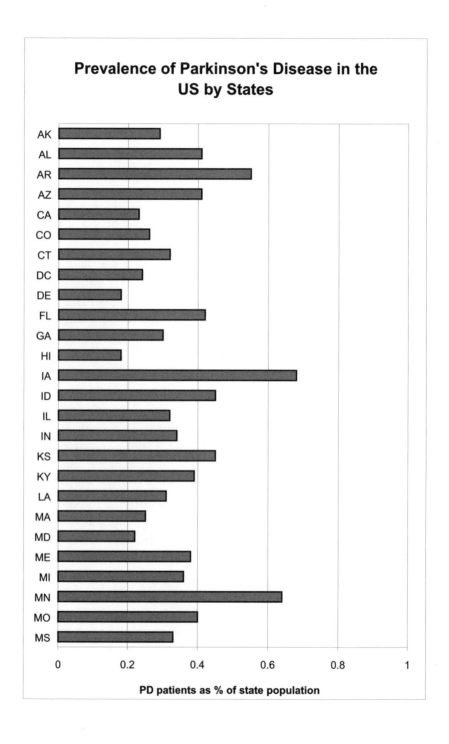

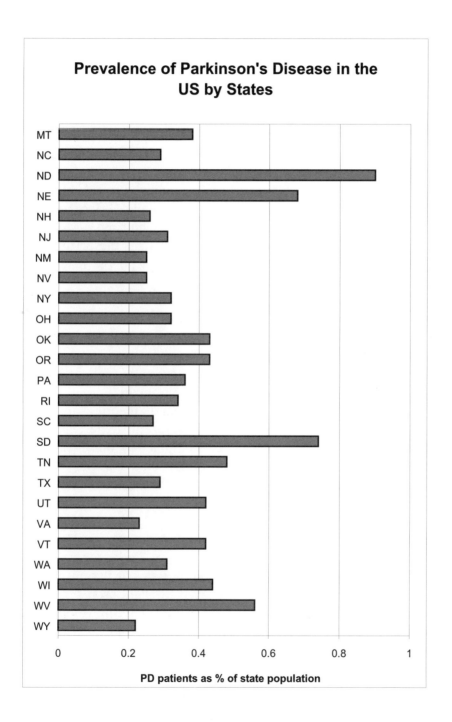

Neurologist Dominique Caparros-Lefebvre noticed that her elderly patients in a hospital in Guadeloupe had the symptoms of ATP. She discovered that many of her patients ate three very common fruits either as solids or in tea form. These fruits are soursop, custard apple, and pomme cannelle. All of these fruits belong to a group of plants from the genus Annonaceae. These fruits have neurotoxic compounds called benzytetrahydroisoquino-line alkaloids.

When Caparros-Lefebvre's patients stopped consuming the fruits, many of them experienced a stabilizing effect in their condition. In some patients, the symptoms disappeared.

Even though many people in the tropics eat these fruits, the neurological problems start to show up when people reach their 60's.

One hypothesis is that children and younger adults may be able to metabolize and excrete neurotoxins more effectively than older adults. Another thought is that it takes a long time for the toxins in the fruit to accumulate to a dangerous level. Along with that is the fact that, as people age, the number of brain cells declines leaving the older population more vulnerable to neurotoxins.

Scientists continue to explore several theories including chemical reactions within the body, exposure to toxic chemicals, genetic factors, and aging. It is possible that any one factor or a combination of factors may cause Parkinson's disease. A more complex theory suggests that along with the combination of environmental toxic exposure, there may also be an inherited inability to rid the body of such toxins, which leads to an increased risk of acquiring PD.

There are many different treatments for Parkinson's disease and its symptoms. There are also different types of Parkinson's. In the previous section I mentioned Atypical Parkinson's. Among people who have Parkinson's, 7% of them have developed the disease from drug treatment. Any dopamine-blocking drug is called a dopamine antagonist and can cause Parkinsonism. Some drugs used to treat high blood pressure like reserpine and methyldopa can cause Parkinson's-type symptoms. So can tranquilizers used to treat psychotic disorders such as schizophrenia. Drug-induced Parkinson's disappears with the cessation of drug therapy.

Exercise Basics

This book addresses the exercise needs of people who have idiopathic Parkinson's disease with symptoms that do not subside, concentrating on the benefits of water exercise.

Most people take water aerobics because their bodies cannot handle the intense impact of land-based exercises, but they still want to exercise and keep fit. As our aging population becomes more concerned with quality of life, they recognize the importance of daily physical exercise in maintaining their health and independence.

A person does not need to become a bodybuilder or a supermodel to reap the benefits of exercise. Most people exercise so they can comfortably perform routine daily tasks such as lifting and carrying children and groceries, doing yard work, or climbing stairs. Our world has become mechanized and convenient and our tasks require less and less physical work. This means that in the future people will have to make a conscious effort to engage in physical activity so their bodies don't lose the ability to perform ordinary daily tasks.

Caregivers or professional fitness instructors who are interested in working with people who have Parkinson's need to be aware of the benefits of basic types of exercises. Older adults and people who have disabilities experience a lack of endurance, strength, balance, and flexibility. These physical conditions can be improved with endurance exercises, strength exercises, and stretching. Endurance exercises are aerobic and improve the health of the heart, lungs, and circulatory system by increasing the heart and breathing rate for extended periods of time. Strength training helps to maintain the integrity of the muscles so they remain strong enough for people to remain mobile and independent. A combination of endurance and strength exercises that focus on posture and walking, along with abdominal exercises, will improve balance and poise thus helping to prevent falls. Stretching keeps the body limber and flexible. All of these basic exercises can be performed easily and comfortably in the water.

Fitness professionals and aquatic instructors know that water is an ideal element in which to work because it envelops all of the submerged joints and limbs and acts as a cushion against jarring motions. Water's buoyancy helps support a person's weight and helps improve balance. Since water is a heavy fluid, the participants are constantly encountering resistance. When a person is in the water, his/her body has a tendency to float. Grounding movements such as walking in the water are the movements that help the body resist the urge to float. This creates more work for the muscles, which in turn strengthens them. As a person moves through the water in all directions, the muscles are being worked on both sides of a joint in a balanced fashion and the muscles are strengthened. The water's pressure helps keep the body's core stabilizers or the torso, in an upright position.

The density of water allows a person to work in a wide variety of planes. These are the vertical or sagittal, the frontal or coronal and the transverse or horizontal plane. The vertical plane divides the body into right and left halves, the frontal plane divides the

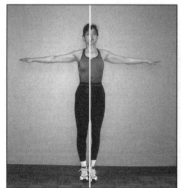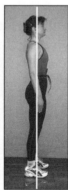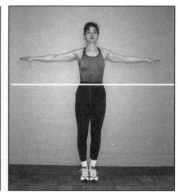

Figure 2. The vertical plane, the frontal plane, and the transverse plane

body into front and back halves, and the horizontal plane divides the body into upper and lower halves. See Figure 2. There are common movements that are done in each of these planes. In the vertical plane, adduction (moving toward the midline) and abduction (moving away from midline) are common movements. In the frontal plane a typical movement would involve flexion and extension. In the horizontal plane, medial and lateral rotation would be typical movements. Working in the water allows the body to move easily in multiple planes.

Moving in water is similar to lifting weights. The more exertion used to move through the water, the more resistance is encountered. This kind of muscle conditioning is different than using weight machines because weight machines stabilize the body except for the muscle group that is being exercised. Weight machines also stabilize the abdominal region while water strengthens the abdominal region in an upright position. This is because this region acts as the body's stabilizing force in the water instead of the body relying on the stabilizing factor of the weight machines. As people start to work in the water, they notice how much their abdominals are used to help them remain upright and balanced in the water while performing various exercises.

In my experience as an instructor at a major health club, I became acquainted with a man who has Parkinson's disease. He was already doing land-based exercises and wanted to add variety to his workouts. We talked about the differences between water workouts and land workouts and agreed that the properties of the water might suit his needs. Before starting any program with him, it was necessary to know what types of exercises were recommended for people with Parkinson's.

The types of exercise recommended for people with Parkinson's are those that help retain the ability of the person to do everyday tasks that are necessary for independent living. Such exercises include retaining mobility and flexibility in the back, shoulders, and neck. Other exercises emphasize leg strength and flexibility to help with reduced balance and postural changes and walking difficulties.

When I learned what those exercises were, I looked to see if there were any kinds of water exercises specific to people with Parkinson's disease. Although I found many exercises recommended for people with Parkinson's that were land-based, I did not find any exercises that were specifically geared towards the water. I took the exercises that were to be done on land and adapted them to the water. Among these are many different types of arm and leg exercises. Walking exercises done in the water provide increased resistance while imitating ordinary movements used in daily living such as pushing a shopping cart, a stroller, or simply walking.

The maintenance of normal muscle tone and function is an important part of the treatment of Parkinson's. With an exercise program specifically designed for the person with Parkinson's, one can learn to compensate for the deficiency of movement caused by the disease thereby greatly improving mobility and independence. If a person finds that skills needed for daily living are improved through specific forms of exercise, then s/he is more likely to keep up with those exercises.

Exercising to enhance posture control, balance, and muscle function is an important part of the therapy used in the treatment of Parkinson's symptoms. W. C. Koller, an expert on Parkinson's Disease, documented that 38% of people living with Parkinson's had fallen and that 13% had fallen more than once a week. In another study, people with Parkinson's suffered fall-related injuries five times more often then healthy adults. This results in an increase in hip fractures with 31% developing complications and dying within three months. As the disease progresses, the propensity to fall increases, due to postural instability and an unnatural response to the center of body mass. Festinating is when a patient freezes in place or walks with a series of small quick steps as if hurrying forward. Festinating causes postural instability. Many who fall do not realize how much of their center of mass has been displaced.

People are more apt to fall when the ratio of their hamstring's strength is less than 2/3 of the strength of quadriceps. This is because, when the quadriceps are stronger, they pull the body forward and off balance. Falls can be lessened by strengthening the ankle joint muscles and flexion at the knee relative to that of the extension. Keeping the leg muscles in the front and back evenly strengthened will help the person with Parkinson's walk with a more balanced gait. A more flexible ankle joint along with a strong, flexible calf muscle will help reduce the shuffling movement common in Parkinson's gait. Exercise improves motor control and functional mobility through walking, range of motion, and flexibility and has been shown to improve and prolong the life of people with Parkinson's.

One of the most debilitating changes a person with Parkinson's experiences is depression. Depression is more common in older patients with Parkinson's than in younger patients. People with Parkinson's and people associated with their care need to be aware of the symptoms and effects of depression. Depression can occur during the course of all chronic illnesses and it is common for people to think that depression is a normal part of chronic illness, but this is not true. Depression is a whole body illness that interferes with work, sleep, appetite, and daily activities.

It is estimated that five percent of the general population suffers from depression. However, 30% to 50% of people with Parkinson's suffer from depression along with at least one third of their caregivers. Many caregivers report that the change in behavior and mood is more stressful than the physical debilitations caused by the disease. Since there are many symptoms of depression that are shared with Parkinson's disease, it can be difficult to detect depression in a person with Parkinson's. These shared symptoms are fatigue, weight changes, loss of appetite, restlessness, sleep disturbance, masked facial expression, and preoccupation with pain or bodily functions.

The symptoms specific to depression are a persistent sad mood, feelings of hopelessness and worthlessness, loss of interest or pleasure in daily living, thoughts of death and suicide, and difficulty with concentration. Often symptoms of depression go undiagnosed because people do not recognize the symptoms or rationalize them as something else; consequently, depression is often overlooked as a serious complication of Parkinson's disease. Dr. Tobias Eichhorn of Philipps University in Marburg, Germany found that depression has more influence on the quality of life among patients with Parkinson disease than the severity of the disease or the side effects of medication.

People with physical disabilities or deformities often suffer from low self-esteem and insecurity about their appearance. They fear they will be rejected by the rest of society for a condition that is beyond their control. Even though their physical appearance and their physical abilities may have deteriorated, they are still the same healthy individual inside that they were before contracting their illness. Exercise helps people suffering from depression, low self-esteem, and insecurity by releasing a class of neurotrans-mitters called endorphins, as well as reducing the levels of the stress-depression hormone, cortisol.

Endorphins are neurotransmitters that are formed in the body by the pituitary gland and act like morphine to relieve pain. Endorphins regulate the contraction of the intestinal wall and help the body to cope with stress, pain, and emotions. Exercise releases endorphins in the body giving the exerciser a euphoric feeling. Exercise also helps a person suffering from depression regain feelings of accomplishment, which leads to improved self-esteem and ultimately a more positive perspective on life.

As you can see, there are many advantages to participating in an exercise program like the one described in *Water Exercises for Parkinson's*. The physical and emotional benefits can be tremendous. As you read through this book and try the exercises, I hope that you will keep working toward health and making the most of your life every day.

1. Exercising

Why Exercise is Beneficial

Exercise is physical activity done with repeated movements in a planned format with the goal of improving physical fitness. A person who has Parkinson's can lead an active lifestyle that includes exercise. Many books on Parkinson's advocate a regular exercise program as part of the daily regime of living with Parkinson's. All too often many formerly active people living with Parkinson's become inactive even when their symptoms are mild, leading to misunderstandings and frustration between the patients and their families and friends.

People with Parkinson's and people who work with them should know the three basic reasons to incorporate an exercise program into the overall treatment of the disease. The first reason is that exercise, as provided by trained professionals or therapists, helps the patients and their families become more familiar and educated about PD. Through this education, the person with Parkinson's and his/her family will better understand what is happening within his/her body and how to work around the limitations of PD. The second reason is that exercise slows down the physical dysfunction associated with PD. In a study done in Germany, 16 people with early to midstage Parkinson's disease did exercises two times a week for 14 weeks. The types of exercise varied from strength training to balancing routines. Afterwards the strength, flexibility, coordination, and walking speeds of the participants were measured. The average strength of the participants increased by 41%, coordination by 42%, flexibility by 21%, and walking speed by 12.5%. The third reason to exercise is to improve the overall fitness level and associated conditioning benefits of the person with Parkinson's.

Many times a person with Parkinson's will stop exercising because of stiff muscles and slowed movement or bradykinesia, which makes exercising more difficult. Dr. James Tetrud of the Parkinson Institute of California has observed that Parkinson's disease does not weaken the muscle itself but, because the disease causes immobility, the muscles become weak and may begin to atrophy due to a lack of use. Regular exercise helps to prevent atrophy and keeps the muscles flexible for a longer period of time. People with Parkinson's need to be encouraged to remain physically active and to maintain a daily exercise program thus avoiding the vicious cycle of less activity leading to loss of muscle tone and strength leading to even less activity. For each day of immobility, there is 1.5% loss of muscle size and endurance and a 5% loss for every three days.

Surprisingly there are differences between men and women who have Parkinson's disease and their willingness to exercise. Rhonda Stanley did a study of exercise intervention in males and females with Parkinson's disease. She found that women, especially those who were sixty-five years and older, resisted the idea of establishing an exercise program. Reasons given by the women were "I can't do that" or "that's too strenuous." Several female participants did not start an exercise program because they did not drive and did not want to impose upon their spouses, relatives, or friends. The females in the study were more willing to suppress their own needs in an effort to appear to be compliant and not be a problem for anyone. This was not the case for the males in the study. The males seemed more willing to take on an exercise program.

Parkinson's disease, as stated before, is a chronic neurologic disease and no amount of exercise will cure it. However, those with Parkinson's disease who stay physically active are able to remain physically independent longer than those who are not active. A study done by Comella, Stebbins, and Brown-Toms compared the physical disabilities of two groups of people with Parkinson's. The clinical trial was done to establish the benefits of exercise as part of the management of Parkinson's. Test subjects were given two hours of rehabilitation exercises three times a week for a period of four weeks. The test group was compared to a control group that did not receive any kind of exercise for the same period. Among the test subjects that exercised, motor function and daily living skills improved dramatically.

Often people with Parkinson's who exercise regularly realize the benefits of their workouts. As the disease progresses they discover they do not have to increase their medication as frequently as those who do not exercise. Some can even decrease their medication. An exercise program should be regarded by people with Parkinson's and their caregivers and physicians as a high priority. It is as important a part of their treatment as the medications they take.

In another study R. Formisano, L. Pratesi, F. T. Modarelli, V. Bonifati, and G. Meco conducted a study that concluded that functional performance of people with Parkinson's improved when physical therapy was used in conjunction with drug therapy. Their research involved two groups of people with Parkinson's that were equally matched with regard to age, severity of symptoms, disease duration, and level of antiparkinson drugs. One group was given only drug therapy and the other group used physical therapy three times a week in one-hour sessions in addition to drug therapy. The study was conducted over a four-month period. At the end of the study, the people with Parkinson's who engaged in physical therapy along with drug therapy showed greater functional improvement in motor performance tests than the group that only received drug therapy.

Exercise programs aimed at people with Parkinson's have traditionally focused on slowing secondary musculoskeletal changes, deconditioning, and the overall deterioration of functional mobility. In a study reported by the *Journal of the American Geriatrics Society*, patients who were in the early to midstage levels of Parkinson's were put on a ten-week exercise routine. The exercises targeted the patient's motor control and gait training. The results showed increased axial mobility, spinal flexibility, and overall physical performance. Another study done by S. S. Palmer, A. J. Mortimer, D. D. Webster, R. Bistevins, and G. L. Dickinson showed patients who exercised using the United Parkinson Foundation exercise program, including a karate program of upper body training, had improved walking gait, better motor control, increased grip strength, and decreased tremors.

Other research supports the position that exercise provides the same benefits to people with Parkinson's as it does to people who do not have Parkinson's. These benefits are increased cardiovascular fitness and muscle strength. Terrie Lee Millard of Temple University did a study of the effects of cardiovascular training on the fitness and motor performance of people with Parkinson's disease. Ms. Millard had sixteen patients with Parkinson's disease who underwent exercise training to measure the effect on participant fitness capacity and secondary motor disability.

The participants were divided into two groups: an exercise group and a non-exercise group. Participants in the exercise group engaged in a three-month aerobic cardiovascular fitness-training program and the non-exercise group engaged in their normal daily activity. The cardiovascular fitness levels of both these groups were measured before and after the three-month study. The group that exercised showed a 34% improvement in their cardiovascular fitness level. These results suggest that cardiovascular fitness greatly affects motor disability and may prolong independence in people with Parkinson's disease.

As mentioned before, many of the water exercises presented in this book are adapted from suggested rehabilitation therapies for people with Parkinson's. Other exercises shown in this book have been adapted from water exercises used to rehabilitate people who have other physical disabilities such as arthritis or who have been injured. Both the people with Parkinson's and the fitness professional or caregiver need to be aware that there is a difference between a person who has been injured and a person with Parkinson's disease.

In the first instance, the person who has been injured started out with a healthy body and hopes to regain that body through rehabilitative exercise. The person with Parkinson's disease started out with a healthy body and is now faced with non-reversible deterioration. The goal for the person with Parkinson's is to use modified exercises to help impede the destructive process of Parkinson's. Instead of seeking an aesthetically pleasing body, the goal of the person with Parkinson's is to remain as independent as possible.

Why Exercising in the Water is Beneficial

Many activities are good forms of exercise. Among them are walking, swimming, running, and biking. However, when people with Parkinson's are given exercises to perform on land, it often causes stress and pain and leads the person to stop exercising. Stiff joints become more rigid and independent movement becomes more difficult. This book, *Water Exercises for Parkinson's,* concentrates on the benefits of walking, stretching, and weight training in the water. The benefits of exercising in the water are numerous and water therapy has been proven to help people with Parkinson's disease.

Water exercises are virtually risk-free. Joints, muscles, and bones are not strained, pulled, or broken due to the cushioning effect of the water. If a person exercises in the water, only 10% of his/her body weight is exerted on the joints, compared to three times the weight when exercising on land. For example, a 100-pound person applies only 10 pounds of pressure on his/her joints when jumping in the water but that same person applies an estimated 300 pounds of pressure on his/her joints when jumping on land. When exercising in water up to the neck, 90% of a person's body is buoyant.

Because of the water's buoyancy, the body's weight is supported, allowing the joints more freedom of movement. The water's support and buoyancy also cuts down on the impact stress to bones and muscles common to land-based exercises. Water's buoyancy allows a person to perform exercises more safely than the same exercises performed on land. Therefore a person with Parkinson's can run, walk, and stretch without risking injury and strain common in land-based exercise programs.

At the Immanuel Rehabilitation Center in Omaha, Nebraska, people with Parkinson's are encouraged to participate in an Aquatic Therapy program. This therapy is based on four principles:

1. Buoyancy: The water's upward thrust acts in opposition to the downward force of gravity. This interaction allows a person to exercise with decreased stress on joints, bones, and muscle.

2. Resistance Force: Water provides resistance to movement in all directions promoting muscle balance and strengthening in antagonists and agonists muscle pairs. Depending on the speed of movement, resistance in the water ranges from 4 to 42 times greater than resistance in the air.

3. Hydrostatic Pressure: Hydrostatic pressure (HP) exerted on the surface areas of an immersed body helps circulate blood from the lower extremities back to the heart. HP increases resistance against the chest forcing the respiratory muscles to work harder and become more developed. HP assistance to the heart helps to lower blood pressure and improve heart rates during water exercises.

4. Warmth: Most therapeutic pools are kept at 93-95°F. The warm water helps relax muscles, reduce joint rigidity, and increase circulation. This allows joints to move through greater range of motion (ROM).

The goals of their Aquatic Therapy Program are

1. Work towards reducing pain.
2. Work towards greater ROM and flexibility.
3. Maintain or improve muscle strength.
4. Regain or improve balance.
5. Maintain or improve cardiorespiratory fitness.

The primary considerations people with Parkinson's have concerning exercise are progressive bradykinesia, rigidity, tremor, and disequilibrium. Bradykinesia means that a person with Parkinson's has significantly slowed and limited movements. Eventually the ability to initiate movement may be lost. Simple daily activities become harder to perform and the rate of performance becomes progressively slower. Rigidity refers to stiffness of the joints and involves all of the limbs. The combination of bradykinesia and rigidity accounts for the symptoms that produce the stooped Parkinson's gait. Swimming and water exercises help to ease the symptoms of bradykinesia and rigidity because the joints and muscles are relieved of stress and strain. Therefore it is easier for the person with Parkinson's to put his/her limbs through a full range of motion.

The most distressing symptom of Parkinson's disease is the tremor. Tremors interfere with the person's ability to engage in voluntary movement and affect mostly the upper body. Water exercises again help to reduce the symptoms of the tremors by allowing the person with Parkinson's to work within an exercise medium that helps the person exert control over his/her muscles. It is easy to move slowly, smoothly, and deliberately through the water because of buoyancy, resistance, and hydrostatic pressure.

Balance is an early problem for a person with Parkinson's. Water is an ideal medium to offset this because the water surrounds the person giving added support. There are many exercises that can be done in the water that can enhance the balance of the person with Parkinson's. Balance is a key factor in daily activities and concentrating on exercises that promote better balance should be a goal of any exercise program.

Some of the exercises that help with a person's balance are

endurance exercises and strength exercises. The endurance (aerobic) exercises that help with balance are The Walk, The Water Jog, The March, The March with a Kick, Crab Walk, Can-Can Kicks, and Heel Kicks. The strength training exercises that help with balance are divided between upper body and lower body. The exercises for the upper body are The Arm Cross, Straight Arm Pulls, Arm Fanning, and Arm Circles. The exercises for the lower body are Squats and Leg Raises both Front and Side. There are also abdominal exercises that help to enhance a person's balance. They are the Standing Front Crunch, Standing Side Crunch, and Trunk Rotation. All of these exercises will be discussed in detail in Chapter 7.

As a person moves through the water and pulls his/her limbs through the water, s/he experiences the resistance of the water. When muscles move, they work in opposing but synchronized pairs. As a muscle contracts the opposing muscle relaxes. The muscles doing the actual work are called the agonists. As the agonists contract, the opposing muscle, the antagonists, relax to allow the movement to continue. In the return move, the roles are reversed. All muscle pairs have a specific ratio of strength to each other. When that ratio is out of balance, possibly due to training of only one of the muscles in a pair, the body works inefficiently and is at risk for injury.

In a person with Parkinson's disease, the balance of opposing muscles is disturbed by the effects of bradykinesia and rigidity. These effects cause the muscles to remain tense and contracted so that a person feels stiff and weak. To get the most effective work-out, it is important to exercise both the agonist and the antagonist muscles. (See Figure 3.) The most important pairs are

- quadriceps/hamstrings
- biceps/triceps
- hip abductors/hip adductors,
- pectoralis major/trapezius and latissimus dorsi
- hip flexor/gluteus
- gastrocnemius/tibialis
- erector spinae/rectus abdominis

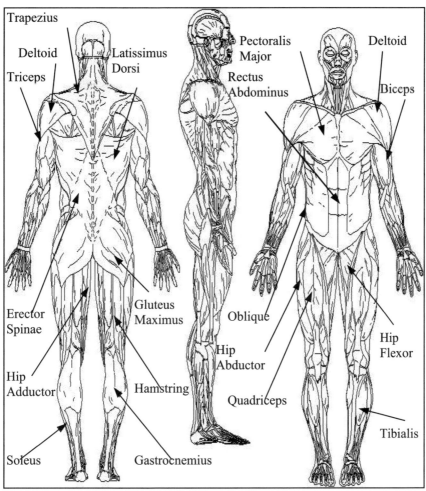

Trapezius

Deltoid

Triceps

Latissimus
Dorsi

Pectoralis
Major

Rectus
Abdominus

Deltoid

Biceps

Erector
Spinae

Hip
Adductor

Gluteus
Maximus

Hamstring

Oblique

Hip
Abductor

Quadriceps

Hip
Flexor

Soleus

Gastrocnemius

Tibialis

Figure 3. Muscle diagram

Exercising in the water causes the muscles to work in pairs. For every muscle that pulls backwards, that muscle's antagonist pulls forward to the starting position. For every upward pull there must be a downward pull. Water increases resistance against the body by an estimated 12% to 14%.

Using the physical properties of water as a fluid alters the intensity of water exercise. Two of these properties are drag and velocity. Drag is the resisting force that opposes movement in the water. Velocity is the speed that an object is moved. When drag is coupled with increased velocity, there is increased water resistance. The resistance of the water is proportional to the velocity needed to move through it. The other properties of water that increase the resistance of water are buoyancy and hydrostatic pressure. Buoyancy is a force that is exerted on a submerged object. An example of buoyant force is demonstrated by holding a Styrofoam dumbbell under the water. Since Styrofoam is lighter than water, the dumbbell wants to move upwards. By using muscles to force the dumbbell to remain underwater the person encounters resistance.

Hydrostatic pressure is force or pressure exerted by water on an immersed body that increases with depth. The pressure also increases with density. Ocean water would exert slightly more hydrostatic pressure than fresh water because ocean water is denser.

Hydrostatic pressure provides equal pressure to the whole body. It helps decrease swelling in the limbs and increases circulation. Hydrostatic pressure does not affect the intensity of water resistance as much as how the body reacts to the intensity of water resistance. Balanced muscles help diminish postural problems. Water resistance allows muscles to move more slowly allowing reaction time to be more deliberate, thus improving balance.

Another added benefit of water exercise is weight control. Aerobic exercise in the water can burn 460 calories an hour. Although land aerobics can burn up to 600 calories an hour, water exercise burns 77% fat calories. Land aerobics burns 43% fat calories. When working in the water, it is easy to achieve both aerobic and anaerobic fitness. Aerobic fitness is achieved through moderate, continuous movement of the large muscle groups for an extended period of time. Anaerobic fitness occurs when a person goes beyond his/her normal endurance level and uses a large amount of energy for a short amount of time.

An example of an exercise that provides both aerobic and anaerobic fitness in water is called Water Walking. Walking through the water at a steady pace for an extended period of time provides aerobic training. Walking in the water at an accelerated pace can push people beyond their aerobic threshold.

Water Walking, when done at a steady pace for 30 minutes can burn as many calories as two hours of land walking. Aerobic training on land can make muscles feel heavy and can put stress on the skeletal system. Anaerobic training on land causes impact to muscles, connective tissues, and weight-bearing joints. Training aerobically in the water avoids the stress and impact of the land, and anaerobic levels can be accomplished because of the water's resistance.

For people who have PD, an aquatic exercise program improves their level of confidence and prolongs their functional independence. When someone is looking for a program that provides all of the necessary exercise modalities in a way that is comfortable for a person with Parkinson's disease, I hope you will agree that exercise in the water just makes sense.

2. Safety in the Water

Parkinson's disease has many different symptoms. While exercise in general, and water exercise in particular, can have many benefits for the person with Parkinson's, it is vital for the person to ask his/her physician for permission before starting any exercise program.

Basics

People with Parkinson's should never swim or exercise in the water alone and only go into a pool when they have a companion or if there is a lifeguard on duty. People with Parkinson's can develop a condition known as "freezing" in which they find their feet and limbs become immobile and seem "frozen" to the ground. If this should occur while they are alone, they can tip forward or backward into the water and be unable to recover. It is very important that the companion working with the participant is able to swim, understands the condition of the patient, and knows CPR. Besides, having another person in the water can make the exercise session a social event, which is even more enjoyable.

Exercise is safer when performed in the shallow end of the pool. All the exercises presented in this book are easy to perform in water that is no higher than chest level. Most of the exercises can be done in water that is waist level. When a person with Parkinson's is exercising in the water, it is advisable for him/her to stay within arm's length of the pool edge just in case freezing or dyskinesia occurs. Should that happen, the exerciser can use the side of the pool to reestablish his/her balance. If the legs feel glued to the ground due to freezing, the toes can be lifted to eliminate the muscle spasm and reestablish movement.

A person with Parkinson's needs to be careful not to over exercise. Over exercising might cause fatigue, which could impair the person's ability to get out of the pool safely. When starting an exercise program, it is important to start slowly and then gradually expand the program. If a person is just beginning an exercise program, s/he should begin with twenty minutes of exercise three times a week, gradually working up to thirty minutes, then forty-five minutes, eventually reaching an hour. This slow build up of exercise duration is important because the person needs to build up endurance or fatigue can set in. This can cause the person with Parkinson's to become frustrated and disillusioned with the program. A good exercise session should leave the person energized rather than tired and frustrated.

Medications

Most people with Parkinson's disease do not start drug therapy until they show functional disability from PD. As Parkinson's progresses, many patients will use medication in addition to exercise therapy to control their symptoms. Long-term use of some drugs can lead to dyskinesia, the uncontrolled, involuntary movement of the face, arms, torso, and legs. Reduced response and fluctuation of motor disabilities is another hazard of long-term drug use. This is why the person with Parkinson's, his/her exercise companion, and the fitness trainer need to have a clear understanding of what medications are being taken, what the desired effects of the medication are, and what the side effects may be, especially how reflexes and response time may be affected.

A variety of medications are used to treat Parkinson's disease. They are divided into three categories: dopamine replacement, anticholinergics, and dopamine agonists. What follows is a list of the most common medications used to reduce the symptoms of Parkinson's disease. The drug name is listed first with the trade name of the drug shown in parentheses.

Levodopa, Carbidopa (Lodosyn®), and Levodopa-Carbidopa (Sinemet® and Atamet®)

The single most effective drug for Parkinson's disease is levodopa. Levodopa converts into dopamine within the brain and compensates for the dopamine deficiency in people with Parkinson's. In order to control the symptoms of Parkinson's disease, patients may require increases in the levodopa medication. Levodopa is a powerful medication and the maximum response time is two to five years. This is called the levodopa honeymoon. While on levodopa, daily performance may change due to a waning effect of the last dose. This waning effect is referred to as the "wearing off phenomenon," and can be lessened by changes in the levodopa dosage. The most common side effect is nausea, but combining levodopa with a carbidopa drug can control the nausea. Different combinations of these drugs are sold under the name Sinemet. Atamet is a frequently prescribed generic equivalent of Sinemet.

One problem associated with levodopa is the "on-off" phenomenon. Patients who exhibit this trait tend to be either completely alert and physically independent or completely immobile and dependent. One minute a person may be ambulatory; a few minutes later s/he may be bedridden. A person with Parkinson's that is affected by the "wearing-off" or the "on-off" phenomena should exercise during an "on" period. Exercising while in an "off" state is dangerous and counter-productive. One medication that helps some is Sinemet CR, which releases medication over a longer time period.

One additional benefit of incorporating exercise into a treatment program is that exercise may increase levodopa absorption. In a study done by Carter, Nutt, and Woodward, ten people with Parkinson's who were taking levodopa engaged in aerobic activity using a stationary bicycle. The participants were given their normal dose of Sinemet and cycled for 35 minutes. Of the ten participants, three showed increased absorption levels of levodopa during exercise, two had no change, and five showed faster levodopa absorption rates after exercise. This study showed that exercise improves levodopa absorption in many people with Parkinson's.

Ropinirole (Requip®)

A new drug has recently been developed called Ropinirole. This drug has the same effect as levodopa but has fewer side effects. In studies done with Ropinirole, patients were four times less likely to develop dyskinesia over long-term use, compared to patients using levodopa. However, levodopa is still the preferred drug to use for the more frail and elderly person with Parkinson's because levodopa has the best immediate efficacy in relation to side effects.

Selegiline (Eldepryl®, Atapryl®, or Carbex®)

Another medication used by people in the early stages of Parkinson's disease is selegiline. The current thought is that the drug helps prolong and enhance the brain's dopamine levels by halting or limiting oxidative processes that injure the cells in the substantia nigra area the brain. The most common side effect is insomnia, so this medication is typically taken with breakfast or lunch.

Pergolide (Permax®), Pramipexole (Mirapex®), and Bromocriptine (Parlodel®) — Dopamine Receptor Agonists

Dopamine receptor agonists (DRA) are synthetic compounds that imitate the dopamine action in the brain. Some dopamine receptor agonists are sold under the names Permax, Mirapex, and

Parlodel. DRA's are used in addition to levodopa. Major side effects of DRA's are nausea, hallucinations, and nightmares. The hallucinations tend to be more of the visual type rather than auditory.

Amantadine (Symmetrel®)

Amantadine is marketed under the name Symmetrel and produces a number of chemical changes in the brain. Amantadine acts as an anticholinergic, helps the brain release dopamine, and simulates neurotransmitters in the basal ganglia area of the brain. Amantadine is used in the early stages of Parkinson's disease before levodopa therapy is started. Amantadine can also be used later in conjunction with levodopa.

The major side effect of Amantadine is livedo reticularis, a benign skin discoloration found mostly in the lower legs. Some people may also experience hallucinations or confusion. If the discoloration from livedo reticularis is a concern to the person with PD, then a long-legged leotard can be worn in the pool. The leotard will keep the legs covered but will not interfere with any activity.

Trihexyphenidyl (Artane®) and Benztropine (Cogentin®)

Other drugs that may have side effects relevant to exercise performance are the anticholinergic drugs such as Artane and Cogentin. In Parkinson's disease, the balance between acetylcholine and dopamine is altered. Acetylcholine is a neurotransmitter that is involved in the transmission of nerve impulses in the body. Anticholinergic drugs decrease the activity of acetylcholine and are effective against rigidity and tremors. The side effects include blurred vision and mental memory impairment. Anticholingics may also exacerbate glaucoma. There are two classes of anticholinergics: piperidyl derivatives and tropanol derivatives. If there are negative side effects with one class of anticholinergics, consult a physician about trying another class.

Beta-Blockers

Beta-blockers such as propranolol, marketed as Inderal®, are agents that help to control tremors that become worse with posture changes or action. Most people with PD use beta-blockers on an infrequent basis. The major side effects of beta-blockers are low blood pressure, slowed heart rate, and depression.

Tolcapone (Tasmar®) and Entacapone (Comtan®) — COMT Inhibitors

There is a new class of drugs called Catechol-O-Methyltransferase inhibitors or COMT. The two drugs in this classification are tolcapone and entacapone. These drugs slow the metabolism of levodopa in the small intestines thus sustaining higher levels of levodopa in the blood for longer periods of time. This increases the time between levodopa doses. Tolcapone is sold under the name Tasmar. Tasmar can increase "on" time by 25% and decrease "off" time by 40%. Unfortunately, Tolcapone has been indicated in several life threatening cases of liver failure and is not used as a first choice medication in the fight against Parkinson's disease

The most common side effects of COMT medications are nausea, drowsiness, dizziness, confusion, dyskinesia, and sleep disorder. Less frequent side effects are headaches, vomiting, constipation, sweating, and urine discoloration. Rare side effects are liver failure, fatal hepatitis, tremor, depression, hallucinations, and adverse drug interaction.

Tricyclic Compounds

These are drugs to help counter the effects of depression. The most commonly used antidepressant drugs for Parkinson's are the tricyclic compounds. Not only do the antidepressant drugs improve the mood of the person with Parkinson's but they also alleviate the symptoms. However, the tricyclic drug side effects include dizziness upon standing, and in patients with heart disease, may cause changes in the heart rhythm. Other side effects of the various medications are confusion, insomnia, changes in mental state, and gastrointestinal upset.

Remacemide Hydrochloride

Another new drug treatment involves using Remacemide Hydrochloride in addition to other dopaminergic drugs such as levodopa. The April 25, 2000, issue of *Neurology* reported on a study using 200 patients with early Parkinson's disease who were not taking any dopamine drugs. Patients received either Remacemide Hydrochloride or a placebo for five weeks. The patients who received Remacemide Hydrochloride were able to complete common daily activities without interference from the symptoms of Parkinson's.

Research has shown that if a neurotransmitter in the brain called glutamate is overactive, a person will exhibit signs of Parkinson's disease. An overactive glutamate neurotransmitter causes excitation of brain cells leading to brain cell death and Parkinson's disease progresses. Remacemide Hydrochloride interferes with glutamate. By interfering with glutamate, Remacemide Hydrochloride seems to be a neuroprotector and may help prevent the progression of Parkinson's disease. The drug has been tested on animal subjects with Parkinson's disease and also has been used in clinical trials for other diseases such as epilepsy, stroke, and Huntington's. Patients in the study reported feeling nausea and dizziness but no other serious side effects.

Clindamycin

Some drug treatments for Parkinson's involve using existing drugs that are prescribed for other conditions. One such drug is clindamycin, which is an antibiotic. Clindamycin has the ability to inhibit nicotinergic transmission. More studies are needed but clindamycin seems to help reduce tremors.

Estrogen

Another existing drug in the treatment of Parkinson's disease is estrogen. Parkinson's disease affects men more often than women. Women who do have Parkinson's are three times more likely to have had a hysterectomy. This suggests that a natural source of estrogen may provide women with some protection against Parkinson's. Women who have Parkinson's but are on hormone replacement therapy (HRT) perform better on basic physical skills tests than women with Parkinson's who are not on HRT. In a study done by the National Institutes of Health, women with Parkinson's who were on HRT were able to absorb the drug levodopa better than women with Parkinson's who were not on HRT. HRT is used to help women with Parkinson's but not men due to estrogen's feminizing side effects.

Clothing

Wearing the proper attire in the water is important for safety. Women and men should both wear swimming suits that fit properly. Besides being uncomfortable, an ill-fitting suit, especially a woman's, will fill with water, adding additional weight. This causes drag and, when the person shifts direction, the drag could cause the exerciser to lose his/her balance. Drag from the water is desirable in an exercise program, but the person engaged in the exercise should have control over the drag force. The swimsuit should not become a drag force. Furthermore, if a person wears a suit that is too tight or small, s/he might experience movement restriction and circulation problems.

When exercising in a pool, it is advisable for the person with Parkinson's to wear water shoes. Many sporting good stores now sell such shoes. The shoes look like other exercise shoes, but they are made to withstand the water and have perforations so the water can easily drain out allowing the shoes to dry more efficiently. Other shoes look more like rubber socks or slippers. See Figure 4.

All are made of water and chlorine resistant material such as neoprene. A person with Parkinson's will want shoes that have Velcro closures, drawstring closures, or shoes that pull on. Shoes add stability and traction in the water, and they protect the tender soles of the feet in and out of the water.

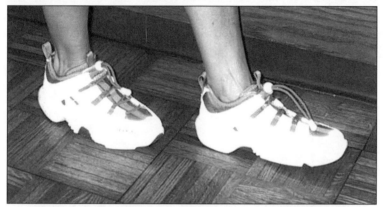

Figure 4. Water shoes with a drawstring closure

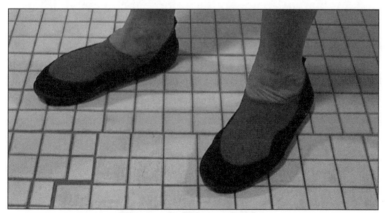

Figure 5. Water Socks

Goggles are optional. Some people are very sensitive to the chlorine levels used in many public and health club pools. Their eyes may become irritated even if they don't submerge their heads under the water. A person who chooses to wear goggles needs to make sure s/he can see clearly out of them. Many goggles are made with lenses that are resistant to fog. Polyvinyl or other soft foam material around the lenses makes the goggles fit snugly against the skin and provides more comfort. Ordinary sunglasses sometimes work just as well.

If the person with Parkinson's and the companion use an outdoor pool, a lightweight T-shirt may be worn for both comfort and protection from the sun. It is important that the T-shirt fit well and not be too loose or else it can get tangled in some of the equipment or cause an unnatural drag effect. It is also advisable to use sunscreen and to wear a hat. A sunburn will interfere with a good workout.

Pools and Their Access

People with disabilities use pools in health clubs and public communities with great regularity and account for 14% of the population that uses pools. Therefore, the method in which a person with Parkinson's is able to enter and exit a pool safely and easily is important.

In 1996, the National Center on Accessibility conducted a Swimming Pool Accessibility study and came up with some pool accessibility recommendations. These are

1. There should be at least one means of accessible water entry/exit.
2. Swimming pools of more than 300 linear feet of pool edge should have two water exit/entries.
3. If only one entry/exit exists, it should be a wet ramp, zero-depth entry, or a lift chair.
4. If a second entry/exit exists, it should be a transfer wall, transfer steps, moveable wall, wet ramp, a lift chair, or zero-depth entry.
5. Wet-ramps, lifts, and zero-depth entry should be used as only one means of entry/exit when other access is available.

6. Both ends and sides of the pool should be served if there are two accessible entry/exits provided.

Besides ordinary stairs, there are five ways a person with Parkinson's can enter a pool safely: lifts, zero-depth entry, transfer walls and steps, dry ramps, and moveable floors. Among people with physical disabilities, lifts, ramps, and zero-depth entry are the preferable methods of pool access.

Lifts

Lifts are plastic chairs or mesh swings that are operated electrically, with water pressure, or with a hand crank. They allow a person to sit down and be transferred in and out of a pool or to transfer from a wheelchair into the lift and be transferred into the pool.

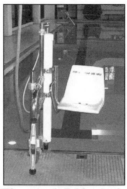

Figure 6. Lift chair

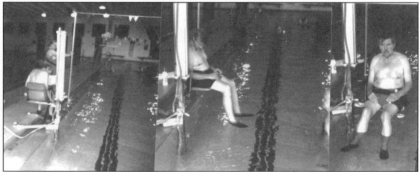

Figure 7. Lift chair in use

Zero-Depth Entry (ZDE)

This is the most popular method of entry/exit by both the general and disabled public. ZDE was originally designed to mimic a beach entry and is used in water-park wave pools. The access starts at deck level or zero-depth, and gradually slopes to the bottom of the pool. This type of pool access is ideal for anyone using an aquatic wheelchair.

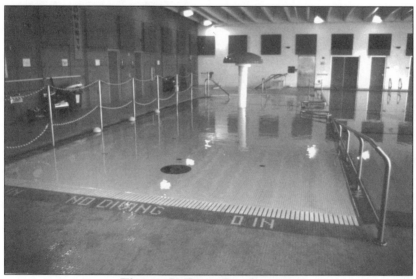

Figure 8. Zero-depth entry

Transfer Walls and Steps

These are raised edge walls or tiers and are used for semi-recessed pools. Transfer walls and/or steps allow a person to transfer from a wheel chair into the pool by grabbing onto the rails and sliding sideways onto the top tier and then lowering himself/herself into the water.

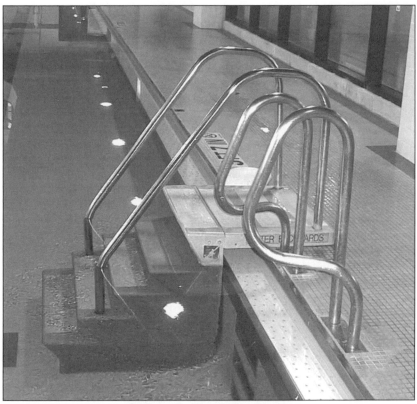

Figure 9. Transfer Steps

Dry Ramps

Dry ramps start at zero-depth and go to a point where the pool transfer wall is elevated. Dry ramps are built into the pool decks and go along the outside of an in-ground pool. They are the easiest and most efficient entry/exit system. They require less space within pool areas and special aquatic wheelchairs are not needed.

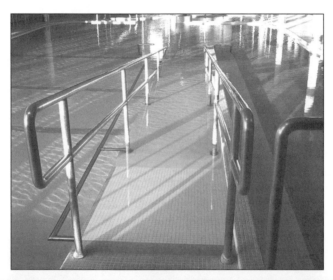

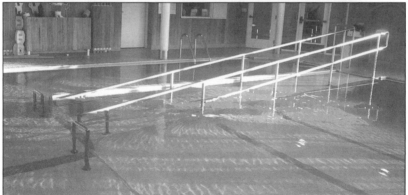

Figure 10. Dry ramps

Moveable Floors

Moveable floors move up and down from zero-depth to maximum depth allowing easy access. The moveable floor is installed over a portion of the pool floor's surface or can cover the entire pool floor. The floor uses a hinged trailing ramp, a vertical elevator, or a rolling bulkhead. A fully raised floor prevents unauthorized pool access, helps pools retain their heat, and prevents evaporation. Even with these advantages the moveable floor is expensive and the least favored method of entry.

When considering what pool or facility to use, keep in mind the ease of entry and exit. People with disabilities such as Parkinson's disease need exercise guidelines, facilities, and equipment that meet their needs. It is one thing to encourage a person with disabilities to exercise and another thing for the person to be able to accomplish the task.

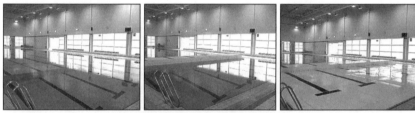

Figure 11. Moveable floor

It is easy for able-bodied people to go to a facility and use the equipment without any trouble, but that is not always the case with people who have Parkinson's disease or other disabilities. Facilities for these people need to be integrated and convenient. Exercise facilities such as those at the YMCA and other health centers that comply with the Americans with Disabilities Act are easily accessible to all groups of people. Since our population is aging, and people with disabilities and limitations are a growing part of the mainstream population, equipment that can be used by all is not only essential but is good business as well.

3. The Exercise Companion

General Overview

This chapter is written for the people involved with the water exercise program: the participant who has Parkinson's and the exercise companion who is in the support role. It is important for the participant and the companion to understand what each other's roles and expectations are. This chapter will help them to work together and forge a productive and effective working relationship. There is one more role that is important in an exercise program, the professional who designs the program. How the professional should assess the participant and design the program is described in Chapter 8, *Designing an Exercise Program.*

Most of the time when people work out together, they do so in order to support and motivate one another. Each person will have his or her own workout. This is not the case for someone who has chosen to work with a participant who has Parkinson's because the participant requires continuous monitoring and evaluation. The partner's role is to be a supportive coach and helper. If the person with Parkinson's has uncontrollable tremors or balance problems, the companion may need to physically support him/her or help him/her to hold onto the equipment. It may be best if the companion is a family member or close friend. It is also possible to hire a fitness professional as a companion.

Whether the companion is a family member, friend, or fitness professional, that person must be informed about the important issues concerning Parkinson's symptoms, treatment, and drug therapies. While the participant's physician and fitness professional will be responsible for the design of the program, knowing the terminology will help the companion to do a better job of helping the participant.

One of the most common ways of describing the abilities of a person with Parkinson's is to use the Hoehn & Yahr stages. The five stages are

1. Unilateral involvement with minimal or no functional impairment.
2. Bilateral involvement or midline involvement without impairment of balance.
3. First sign of impaired righting reflexes evident by unsteadiness as the patient turns or is pushed from standing equilibrium with feet together and eyes closed.
4. Fully developed, person is severely disabled; but is still able to walk and stand without assistance although is markedly incapacitated.
5. Confined to bed or wheelchair, no movement unless assisted.

Other assessment rating tools are the UPDRS (Unified Parkinson Disease Rating Scale) and the Schwab and England Activities of Daily Living Assessment.

The UPDRS is divided into three sections. The first section evaluates mental abilities, behavior, and mood. The second section rates the level of daily activities and the third section evaluates motor skills. The three sections are broken down by ratings of zero to four with zero representing the most independent and four indicating total dependency. For the scale as a whole there are a possible 199 points with 199 being the most impaired.

The Schwab and England evaluation is done by percentages. A rating of 100% means the person with Parkinson's is completely independent. A zero percentage rating means the person with

Parkinson's is totally dependent upon others for all of his/her needs and is bedridden. The scale is broken down by percentage points and each decline of 10% represents another, more advanced level of Parkinson's disease. The UPDRS and The Schwab and England Activities of Daily Living are used more by professionals and will be examined in detail in Chapter 8. Of all the scales used to measure the progression of Parkinson's disease, the Hoehn & Yahr scale is the most common. It is also the easiest to use to assess the abilities of people with Parkinson's, as well as those who are assisting with an exercise program. More details on these scales are available on the web from the Functional and Stereotactic Neurosurgery Department of the Massachusetts General Hospital at http://neurosurgery.mgh.harvard.edu/pdstages.htm.

There are other points to consider when designing an exercise program for the person with Parkinson's. The companion needs to learn which exercises help the participant maintain balance, posture, strength, and endurance and how to help the person with Parkinson's execute these exercises effectively. It is also important for the companion to understand that these exercises will enable the person with Parkinson's to improve his/her ability to perform activities of daily living. As Parkinson's disease progresses, especially if there is mental degeneration, increased physical and verbal cueing may be needed. The companion should be aware that the program might need to be modified from time to time to continuously meet the changing needs of the person with Parkinson's.

When helping with an exercise program, the companion must address:

- stretching involving relaxation
- balance and upright posture
- respiratory ability
- general flexibility or range of motion (ROM)

An exercise program should therefore consist of cardiovascular training, flexibility training, and strength training. The companion needs to assess if the person with Parkinson's can stretch effectively and determine if s/he is flexible and strong enough to engage in strength training and flexibility training. The exercise program should have elements that address each of these areas and the companion's role is to ensure that these areas are addressed in the exercises actually performed by the participant.

Relaxation is important as a way to reduce problems with muscle rigidity. Exercises that help induce relaxation include stretching and deep breathing.

Postural maintenance or balance is important because maintaining upright posture helps people with Parkinson's maintain balance and allows them to move and walk more efficiently. Postural maintenance also helps respiratory capacity and aerobic ability. Stooped posture inhibits the diaphragm, which needs to expand in order to breathe properly. Some of the exercises that help with postural maintenance include Heel Kicks, Crab Walk, and Arm Cross.

Respiratory capacity refers to the ability to endure aerobic activity. Exercises that help with respiratory capacity include The Water Walk, March with a Kick, and any of the aerobic exercises found in Chapter 7. Other exercises that are helpful with respiratory capacity include the back and pectoral stretches found in Chapter 6 and trunk rotation found in Chapter 7.

Flexibility training concentrates on increasing range of motion (ROM). Range of motion is important because improving ROM improves fluidity of movement. Flexibility combats stiffness and muscle atrophy. Some of the exercises that help with ROM are leg raises, arm raises, trunk rotation, and neck rotation. These can be found in Chapter 7.

How to be an Exercise Companion

The primary goal of the exercise companion is to help promote the physical and emotional independence of the participant in the exercise program. A companion does not need to be a fitness professional in order to be an effective companion to someone with Parkinson's. The companion does need to become knowledgeable about Parkinson's and the types of exercises that are beneficial to people with Parkinson's. This book, *Water Exercises for Parkinson's*, is written so both professionals and non-professionals can work with those who have Parkinson's.

If the companion is a friend or family member, s/he may want to be coached by a fitness professional before working with the person with Parkinson's. A good way for the layperson to understand the exercises and the benefit of the exercises is to perform the exercises while the fitness instructor plays the role of the companion. Once the companion becomes familiar with the exercises, it will be easier to guide the participant through them. For practice, the companion can guide the fitness instructor through the exercises and make sure that s/he understands the benefits of each exercise and how they should be executed. After the companion has experienced both sides of the partnership, s/he will be better able to assist the person with Parkinson's.

It is best for the person with Parkinson's to have a consistent companion rather than a series of companions so intimate nuances in communication, both verbal and non-verbal, are understood and stay consistent. The companion has to be sensitive to the physical and emotional changes in the person with Parkinson's due to medication and/or the progression of the disease.

When the disease reaches a more advanced stage, the companion will have to use constant visual and verbal cueing. The companion must be wary of becoming frustrated with having to cue and re-cue a person with failing skills. The goal is to encourage mental and physical function at as independent a level as possible. If the companion becomes frustrated with the difference in ability between himself/herself and the participant, the companion may be tempted to gloss over the exercises or omit them altogether to save time.

As Parkinson's disease progresses, it may become necessary for the person with Parkinson's to be assisted by two companions. One partner can help cue and guide the participant through the exercises and the other companion can concentrate on keeping the participant balanced and stable. The reward for being the companion is the prolonged and improved life of the person s/he assists, especially if the companion is a family member.

Whether the companion is a family member, friend, or professional, it is his/her responsibility to encourage the person with Parkinson's to perform the exercises correctly. This includes ensuring that the person with Parkinson's keeps his/her head up with the chin parallel to the floor, that s/he fully extends the arms in a natural swinging motion, and that s/he does not shuffle.

Throughout the exercises, the companion should monitor the patient for signs of fatigue and give frequent verbal encouragement. Statements such as "that's great," "you're doing well," or "you're doing better" reinforced with physical corrections such as a gentle lift of the participant's head when it drops forward or a guiding touch on the shoulder to direct the participant through a movement is important. The companion should never force a muscle or joint to move but should allow the person to do as much as possible on his/her own. The physical touch by the companion not only helps the person with Parkinson's stay poised and balanced but also assures the person that s/he is accepted as s/he is. Exercising for the person with Parkinson's is not only valuable for the physical benefits but also for the companionship and support that comes from working and socializing with other people.

Exercising with a person with Parkinson's is much different than exercising with a person without Parkinson's. People with Parkinson's have special needs because of their disability and they do better in sessions that are private with one-on-one instruction versus a group setting, especially as the disease progresses. In order to be an effective instructional partner, it is important to plan workouts carefully, present the exercises clearly and with demonstrations, manage time effectively, individualize the program, give positive feedback, and prepare for the unexpected.

When planning a workout for a person with Parkinson's, his/her individual needs must be considered first. People with Parkinson's have a heterogeneous syndrome, which means they must deal with several dissimilar disabilities all at once. Depending on the stage of the disease, the time and amount of medication, exercise performance will vary, sometimes in a very short time. This becomes a challenge to the companion because performance expectations for the person with Parkinson's will have to be adjusted. Some days the person with Parkinson's will do poorly and other days s/he will excel. Under these conditions, patience is a must as well as a virtue.

The way information is presented to a person with Parkinson's can make the difference between an effective, enjoyable workout and an unpleasant experience. Exercise partners must give clear directions about what they are teaching and why. It is not enough to instruct a person with Parkinson's how to do the Water Walk; s/he also needs to know that the Water Walk will help gait and balance. Demonstrating a desired exercise is essential. Visual cues with the hands and legs along with verbal instruction tend to be more effective than verbal cues alone. The instructor or partner should be sure the participant understands the exercise. The instructor needs to initiate feedback from the person with Parkinson's about how s/he is doing.

Time management is an important aspect of the exercise routine. Since people with Parkinson's tire easily, they need to exercise while still fresh and alert. To prevent waiting time, routines and equipment should be ready prior to the start of an exercise session. Giving clear cues also cuts down on repeated instructions thus keeping the exercise routine running smoothly.

Each person with Parkinson's must be assessed individually. Since different stages of the disease require different levels of guidance and instruction, exercise programs must be tailored to each individual. The level of ability of a person with Parkinson's will determine the amount of physical and verbal cueing done by the companion or instructor. Throughout the exercise session, the partner or instructor needs to be enthusiastic and provide encouragement.

One of the most difficult situations a companion or instructor can face is when the person with Parkinson's freezes. When a person freezes, s/he becomes immobile. S/he may also be unaware that s/he is frozen. If the companion or exercise instructor is unfamiliar with this phenomenon, s/he may view this behavior as obstinate and rude. Often having the participant step over an imaginary object on the pool floor will break the neurological immobility. If the person with Parkinson's freezes, the companion can encourage him/her to either reach out or step over an imaginary object. The instructor can also place his/her foot out in front of the participant so s/he can step over it. Marching in place works for some people and loud sudden noises, such as clapping, work for others.

A summary of cueing techniques:

1. Use metaphors, similes, and imagery. Examples would be to say "stand as straight as an arrow," "walk like a soldier," "kick as if a ball is in front of you."

2. The instructor or partner can be a visual cue. Examples would be to tell the person with Parkinson's "put your arms out to the side like me" or "look at what I am doing."

3. Question the person with Parkinson's to establish feedback and communication. Examples: "Can you feel the muscle working?" "Are you comfortable being in deeper water?"

4. The instructor, partner, or companion needs to show empathy. Let the person with Parkinson's know his/her efforts are appreciated. Phrases like "I know this is hard" or "I know this is the best you can do" are good examples.

5. Establish a positive bond by engaging in conversation before and after the exercise session. After a trusting relationship has been developed between the person with Parkinson's and a partner or instructor, humor can be used as a cueing tool during instruction. Humor helps to establish a more unique and personal bond.

6. Verbal feedback should be positive and specific. If the person with Parkinson's has performed a routine well, s/he needs to be told specifically what was done and why it is beneficial. Instead of saying "good work," say "you are walking much better and you are picking up your feet."

7. Kinesthetic feedback is feedback concerning physical

contact. Physical cueing is very useful when working with an exerciser during a strength training session. An example would be to help the person with Parkinson's execute an exercise by physically touching the body part that is to be moved such as an arm, and guiding the arm through the desired motion.

Seniors Working Together

Parkinson's affects mostly seniors and many seniors live in their own communities. Many of these communities are in warm climates that have swimming pools, so it is likely that the companion to the person with Parkinson's will also be a senior. More than likely, this person will be a spouse or close friend. This presents unique challenges for both people. While one person is coping with Parkinson's disease, the other person may be coping with arthritis or another age-related condition. It is also possible that the couple working together may both have Parkinson's disease. A person with Parkinson's who is in stage 1 of the Hoehn and Yahr Scale may be quite capable of assisting someone else who is farther along in the disease. In such a case, both members of the team benefit from the exercises. This type of partnership offers a unique opportunity for the pair to offer each other mutual support and encouragement.

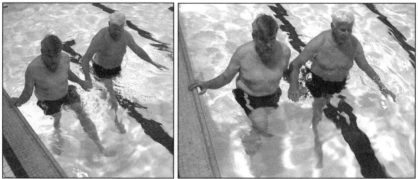

Figure 12. Seniors working together using the pool wall

The person with Parkinson's may feel more comfortable working with someone from his/her peer group. Even though the companion may not be dealing with Parkinson's disease, the fact that s/he may have other age-related concerns could help the couple forge a mutual understanding and empathetic relationship. Given their stage in life, they may have patience for each other in a more natural manner.

While the companionship of one senior helping another may be beneficial in many ways, there are also risks involved that both people must be aware of. A person who suffers from arthritis may not have the reflexes, strength, or flexibility needed to support or lift another person, especially if that person has problems with balance. Likewise, the person with Parkinson's has his/her own issues without having to be responsible for the safety of someone else.

Given the limitations of both people it would be prudent to involve a second companion who is knowledgeable and physically able to assist the two seniors. If a third person is not available, the two seniors would be wise to exercise at a pool or facility that has a lifeguard and inform the lifeguard as to what they are doing.

If another person is able to assist the two seniors, s/he needs to be aware of the limitations of both participants, not just the one with Parkinson's disease. The person with Parkinson's and his/her senior companion will want to enlist the help of a professional fitness instructor before going off on their own. The fitness instructor will assess the physical abilities of both people. The instructor must have a working knowledge of Parkinson's disease and other geriatric conditions such as heart disease, arthritis, diabetes, etc. This will enable the instructor to help each person in the partnership become more aware of his/her capabilities and limitations.

I have worked with a man who has Parkinson's and is between stage 3 and stage 4 of the disease according to the Hoehn and Yahr scale. When he leaves cold and snowy Minnesota in the winter for warm, sunny Florida, he stays in a facility for seniors that has a pool. He travels with a friend who is eighty and has arthritis. They like to work together in the water. I have instructed both of them by teaching Osmund, the companion, what Tom, the person with Parkinson's, did for his exercise routines.

It is important for the senior companion to know how to guide the person with Parkinson's through the exercises without compromising his/her own safety. For Osmund this meant that he and Tom needed to stay within arms reach of the pool wall and not go deeper than mid-chest while performing the exercises. Osmund also needed to become more familiar with the details of Parkinson's and its effects. Tom also became more sensitive to Osmund's arthritis and the balance, flexibility, and strength problems that go along with it. Both men learned that the best exercises for them to perform were the ones involving upright posture or exercises performed near the edge of the pool. These exercises are presented in this book.

Using resistance equipment can also involve risk for people who have balance problems. The person with Parkinson's and the senior companion can use resistance equipment at the same time only as long as the pool wall supports both of them.

4. Equipment

As the participant progresses in the water exercise program, s/he should plan to supplement the natural resistance of the water with resistance equipment. These are available as: gloves, water weights, paddles, ankle weights, noodles, kickboards, and jogging belts. All of this equipment can be purchased from fitness stores or can be ordered through the Internet. Many health clubs and rehabilitation centers have some or all of these items and will generally allow people to use them. A description of this equipment follows.

Water Gloves

Water gloves are made of neoprene or chlorine resistant Lycra and have webbing between the fingers. This allows the hands to grab, push, or pull more water and thereby gain more resistance and intensity. The gloves are easy to put on, easy to remove, and have a Velcro clasp at the wrist. These are especially good for people who have a trouble holding onto free weights.

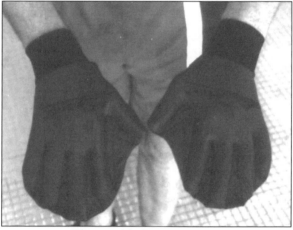

Figure 13. Water gloves

Water Weights

Water weights look like dumbbells or barbells but are made of Styrofoam plates and a plastic bar. More expensive models use closed cell EVA foam. These are more durable than Styrofoam and the plates are non-abrasive. The bar between the plates is padded to help reduce over gripping. Dumbbells are held in each hand and barbells are held with both hands. Barbells are 25"-30" in length. Some barbells have a curved bar to allow for better hand positioning. Dumbbells and barbells come in varying weights and sizes. Both are feather light on land but are resistant to water since Styrofoam is buoyant. By manipulating the dumbbells under water, the user gains the same level of resistance training that a weight trainer has when using metal dumbbells on land. The dumbbells and barbells are used mostly to help strengthen the upper body, arms, chest, torso, and back.

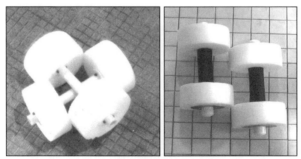

Figure 14. Water weights

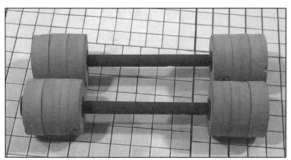

Figure 15. Water barbells

Paddles

Paddles are plastic dumbbells that have pinwheels at the ends instead of Styrofoam plates. The paddles provide resistance when dragged through the water. The pinwheels are adjustable. The pinwheels can be opened for less resistance, allowing water to flow through the wheel, or closed, allowing for more resistance. It is advisable to start with the paddles before progressing to the water weights or noodles.

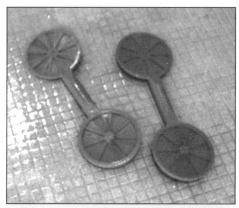

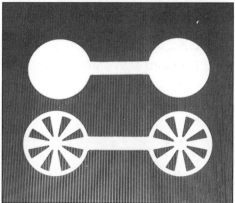

Figure 16. Water paddles

Ankle Weights and Water Wings

Ankle weights and water wings are cuffs made for both the wrist and the ankle. They are made of soft Santoprene rubber or nylon covered Styrofoam. They provide both drag and buoyant resistance like water weights. Since they are strapped onto the body, it is easier to have control of them versus water weights. For the beginner who may not be used to any type of water equipment, it might be easier to start with ankle weights, water wings, or paddles. Once these pieces of equipment have been mastered, then the person can attempt water weights.

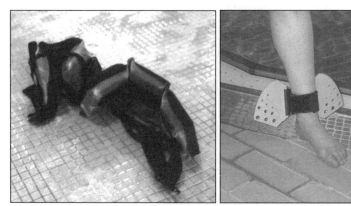

Figure 17. Ankle weights and water wings

Noodles

Noodles are long cylindrical tubes made of Styrofoam. They were originally made as flotation toys for children. There are two types of noodles, one is hollow and the other is a solid tube. The hollow tube is easier to manipulate. Both kinds come in varying lengths. Again, by manipulating the Styrofoam tube underwater, the user is able to increase the water resistance. The noodles are used for strengthening the legs, abdominal work, and to stabilize and enhance a person's balance.

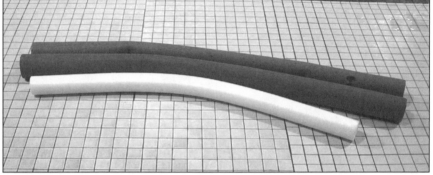

Figure 18. Noodles

Kickboards

Kickboards are buoyant, durable, lightweight flat boards that can be used to help a person support himself/herself in the water while performing exercises. The most common type of exercise that uses a kick board is one where a person is prone in the water.

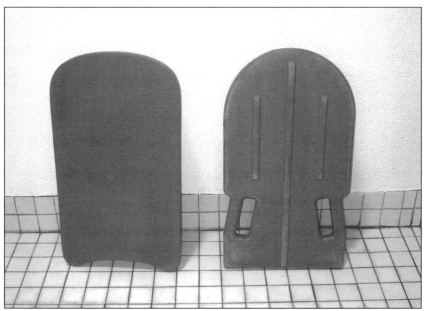

Figure 19. Kickboards

Jogging Belt

The jogging belt is used to raise the body from the floor of the pool and maintain a person in a vertical position. The belts come in different styles. Some are wide, sculpted EVA type foam belts and others are made of foam blocks that are strung on a nylon belt. The wide, sculpted belts are more expensive and offer a little more security.

The jogging belt can be used in water as shallow as chest deep. This is a helpful piece of equipment for a person with sore knees, ankles, or feet. The belt relieves those joints of the body's weight while still allowing for freedom of movement to run, jog, or bicycle in the water. It is very important to understand that the jogging belt is not a flotation device and should never be used as such.

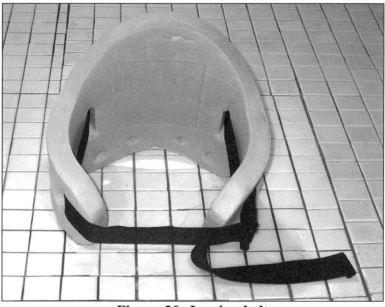

Figure 20. Jogging belt

Equipment for Advanced Parkinson's

Other types of equipment may be needed as Parkinson's progresses. These are a cane, a walker, an aquatic wheelchair, a stool, and a lift chair. A cane or walker made of water-resistant material can withstand the water and gives the person a better sense of balance and security. These also help provide extra stability for episodes of "freezing." The person with Parkinson's should not correct stooped posture by having a cane or walker that is too high. This could cause balance instability and result in falling backwards. A stool can be used when standing or walking in the water becomes too difficult. The person with Parkinson's can do many arm and leg exercises in a seated position. An aquatic wheelchair consists of a frame made of plastic, hollow tubes, and water-resistant canvas. Most pool facilities that specialize in programs for people with physical limitations provide aquatic wheelchairs. A lift chair is a moving, motorized chair found at pools that are in hospitals and other rehabilitative centers. These chairs are used to help people get in and out of the water. They are used by people who have little to no ability to walk.

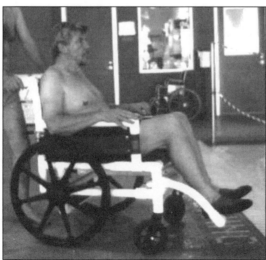

Figure 21. Water wheelchair

5. Preparing to Exercise

An exercise program consists of three main components: cardiovascular training (CV), flexibility training (FT), and strength training (ST).

In order for the person with Parkinson's to get the optimum benefits of water exercises it is important for the participant and the companion to follow guidelines for people with Parkinson's. The following recommendations are from the National Parkinson Foundation, and are designed to stimulate all of the major muscle groups.

1. The person with Parkinson's needs to plan 15-20 minutes of actual exercise time each day. In addition s/he needs to set aside enough time to dress, arrive at the exercise location, warm up and cool down, and clean up and refresh himself/herself. The actual time for the entire procedure will vary from one to two hours. Actual exercise time can be increased depending on the participant's strength level, medications, and physical endurance.

2. The person with Parkinson's should take at least five minutes to warm up before doing any exercises. These warm-ups may be a mix of gentle stretching and slow stationary movements for the arms and legs. Warming up properly encourages blood flow to the muscles and helps to prevent injuries.

3. The person with Parkinson's should try to perform each exercise correctly to its full potential. The partner or fitness trainer will be able to help the person with Parkinson's by monitoring his/her progress through effective, positive visual and verbal cueing. Throughout the warm-ups, stretching, and exercise

portions of the exercise routine, the companion should give visual and verbal cues.

4. Before increasing the intensity or repetitions of any of the exercises, the person with Parkinson's should have performed the exercises at a constant level for 4 to 5 days. After that time frame, if the person with Parkinson's feels the exercises are less demanding and can be performed without difficulty, s/he may want the challenge of increased intensity or repetitions.

5. It is not only important to stretch before an exercise session; stretching is essential to maintaining and improving flexibility. In addition to stretching, the person with Parkinson's should do some deep breathing exercises after each session.

After exercising, the person with Parkinson's will need to relax. This is time set aside for personal physical and mental improvement. Many people feel if they take the time to indulge in self-improvement, they are being selfish and neglecting other people in their families. This may be because other family members project such an attitude. The word "indulge" is appropriate because that is how some people feel about self-improvement.

In the study previously described, and undertaken by Rhonda Stanely, the women participants didn't want to impose on family members. They viewed their need to exercise as an indulgence and an imposition on their families. Unfortunately, the women's feelings were not addressed.

The person with Parkinson's must not feel guilty or be made to feel guilty for engaging in self-improvement. If a person is not as healthy as s/he can be, both inside and out, and if s/he feels s/he is not in control of his/her destiny, or an active part in his/her destiny, s/he may become a burden to himself/herself and other family members and friends. One of the most important aspects of preparing to exercise is understanding that it is worth the time and effort.

6. Warm-Ups and Stretching

Warm-Ups

The participant and the companion should take at least five minutes to warm up before doing any exercises. There are several warm-ups described in this chapter. Generally warm-ups should emphasize the lower body before the upper body. They may include slow stationary movements for the legs and arms and a mix of gentle stretching. Warming up properly encourages blood flow to the muscles and helps to prevent injuries.

There are five good overall warm-ups to be done in the water. They are the Water Cycle, Water Jog, Walking, The March, and The March with a Kick. These warm-ups work the entire body, specifically the feet, ankles, thighs, hips, buttocks, back, shoulders, wrists, and arms.

Water Cycle

For this warm-up, the person uses a jogging belt and is in water deep enough so his/her feet do not touch the bottom when wearing the jogging belt. If there is not a jogging belt available or the person with Parkinson's does not want to use one, the Water Cycle can be modified to a Water Jog (described in the next warm-up). The belt should be put on before entering the pool. The companion should help the person with Parkinson's put on the belt and make sure it is secured, especially if the person with Parkinson's is experiencing tremors. The parts of the body being warmed up are the shoulders, arms, wrist, chest, back, buttocks, legs, and feet.

Once in a comfortable level of water, the participant can gently move his/her legs in a cycling motion and swing the arms back and forth as if running slowly. The companion should be within arm's reach of the person with Parkinson's in case the participant needs added balance.

The hands should be held in a cupped position. When the hands are cupped, they are able to "grab" water, which adds more resistance. Consider a person putting a hand out of a car window as the car moves down the road. When the fingers are open, the air goes through and it is easy to hold the arm up. A cupped hand makes a sail, and it is harder to hold the arm up because of wind resistance. This is also what water gloves do but, if gloves are not available, cupping the hands is the next best thing.

During the warming up, the companion can verbally and

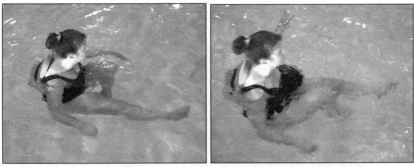

Figure 22. The Water Cycle using a jogging belt

visually cue the person with Parkinson's by making sure the participant has cupped hands, is holding his/her trunk fully upright, and is moving the legs and arms in even smooth strokes. It is important for the companion to give positive reinforcement and encouragement. Do this warm-up or one of the variations that follow for 3-5 minutes.

The Water Cycle can also be done from the side of the pool. See Figure 23. Rest the arms on the edge of the pool and let the legs float out from the sides, then move the legs in a cycling motion. When the Water Cycle is done in this position, only the legs and buttocks are being warmed up. The arms provide leverage to help keep the person upright and stable. Again the companion should be close by in case the person with Parkinson's needs added assistance.

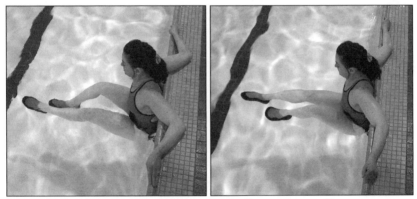

Figure 23. Water Cycle from the wall

If it is too difficult to lean on the edge of the pool, the person with Parkinson's can use a noodle as support by wrapping it around the body and lying on the noodle in a reclining fashion. The companion will need to stand behind the person and hold the noodle from behind. See Figure 24. This will make it easier to hold the head up. The body parts that are being warmed up are the buttocks, the legs, and the feet. While moving, the person with Parkinson's needs to concentrate on holding the body upright to keep from bending forward at the waist. The companion can assist by gently repositioning the person's body when needed as well as verbally cueing the movement of the legs and giving positive encouragement.

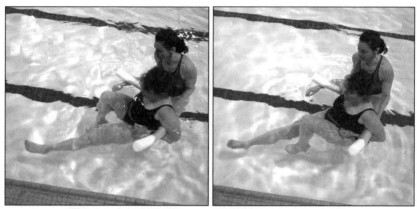

Figure 24. The Water Cycle using a noodle

Water Jog

To do the water jog, the person with Parkinson's and the partner will need to stand in chest-deep water. The parts of the body that are being warmed up are the shoulders, arms, chest, back, buttocks, legs, and feet. The person with Parkinson's should stand close enough to the pool wall so s/he can use the wall for support and balance. For further stability, the person with Parkinson's may want put his/her back against the wall and arms

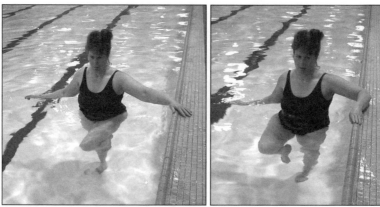

Figure 25. Water Jog

on the pool ledge. (See Figure 26.) With this variation only the buttocks, thighs, calves, and feet are being warmed up. The participant runs slowly in place or in a small circle swinging the arms back and forth in sync with the jogging. When performing the Water Jog, the feet touch the bottom of the pool. With each shift of the foot, the person is propelled slightly upwards. The companion can cue the person with Parkinson's verbally to bring the knees up as high as possible and to try to keep the head up and eyes forward. The companion can also cue the person to move the arms back and forth with cupped hands to their full range of motion. The companion can perform the Water Jog along with the person with Parkinson's thus providing visual cueing and encouragement. Do this warm-up for 3-5 minutes.

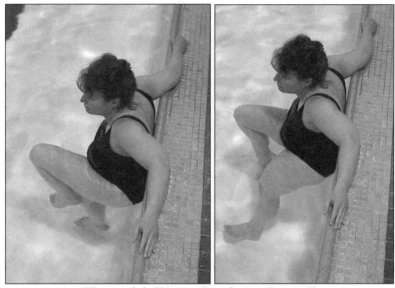

Figure 26. Water Jog from the wall

Water Walk

Standing in chest-deep water, the person with Parkinson's walks a short distance back and forth or in a small circle making sure to swing the arms from the shoulders. The Water Walk can also be done with the assistance of a companion and the participant may want to use the pool edge for added balance. The parts of the body being warmed up are the shoulders, arms, chest, back, hips, legs, and feet. When working with a companion, the person with Parkinson's should position himself/herself between the pool wall and the companion. This allows the participant to hold both the wall and the companion's hand for the most support. While the companion walks with the person with Parkinson's, the companion should cue the participant to hold the head up and to look straight ahead. Also the partner can cue for walking in a heel to toe fashion and monitor for a shuffling gait. The partner should perform the Water Walk along with the person with Parkinson's in order to provide good visual cueing. It is important to take the time to perform the Water Walk correctly rather than to rush through and omit fine points. The partner can also hold the person's hand and guide him/her in a proper arm swing. Do this for 3-5 minutes.

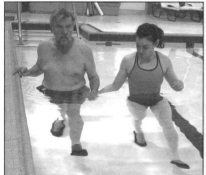 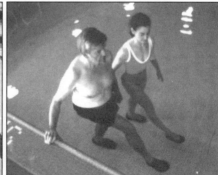

Figure 27. Water Walk

The March

While standing in waist to chest deep water, the person with Parkinson's raises the knee to hip level, then lowers the leg, and repeats the exercise with the other leg. The March is done as an in-place warm-up. The body areas that are being warmed up are the hips, buttocks, thighs, and calves. While the person with Parkinson's performs The March, the companion can stand in front and hold the participant's hands at waist level and encourage the participant to the touch the palms of the hands with the knees. The companion needs to watch for forward leaning and/or sideways tilting. If such posture is noticed, cue the person with Parkinson's to stand upright with the chin up and to look straight ahead. Another place for the companion to be positioned is so the person with Parkinson's is between him/her and the pool wall. The companion can then perform The March along side of the participant. This warm-up exercise needs to be done for 3-5 minutes.

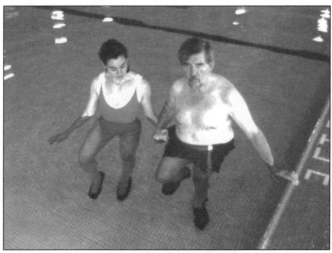

Figure 28. The March

March With a Kick

While standing in water waist to chest deep beside the pool wall, the participant marches in place as in the previous warm-up, but adds a kick. The knee is brought to hip level then the lower leg is extended outward. After returning the straightened leg to the pool bottom, the person with Parkinson's repeats the exercise with the other leg. This warm-up affects the hips, buttocks, thighs, and calves. The companion can stand on the other side of the participant and perform the March with a Kick as a means of visual cueing. The companion can hold the hand of the participant with one hand. The other hand can be used to indicate how high the knee should come and how far the lower leg should stretch out and up. Encourage the person with Parkinson's to keep the torso upright, chin up, and eyes forward. This warm-up exercise is done for 3-5 minutes.

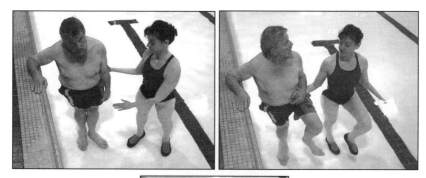

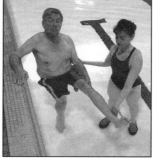

Figure 29. March with a kick

Standing Tall

This warm-up is particularly good for people with Parkinson's. It is designed to help them focus on posture. In shoulder-deep water the person with Parkinson's presses the back, head, shoulders, buttocks, and heels against the wall. Once s/he is stabilized against the wall, the person takes one step forward keeping his/her posture upright. The companion usually assists the person with Parkinson's. When the step is completed, the person takes one step back to return to the wall. The person with Parkinson's should recheck his/her position with any needed help from the companion before taking the next step with the other leg. This warm-up exercise should be repeated with 5-10 repetitions on each leg.

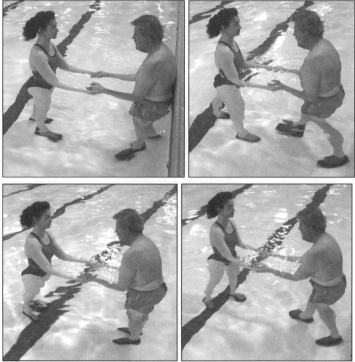

Figure 30. Standing Tall

Stretching

Although stretching is as important to the participant as warming up, it should be approached as a relaxing, pleasant part of the workout session. To avoid pain during stretching, the person with Parkinson's should accept the companion's assistance for the most effective position. With continued stretching, flexibility will increase. Stretching helps to reduce stiffness and soreness that may be caused by working out. Stretching in water is more comfortable and much easier than on land because the water helps the person with Parkinson's keep his/her balance.

How to Stretch

While stretching the person with Parkinson's should:

a. Move slowly and not bounce. Moving slowly through a stretch overrides the reflex reaction and increases the elasticity of the muscles. Bouncing while stretching may cause muscles to tighten instead of loosen and could result in a pulled muscle.

b. Stretch to a point of mild muscle tension and not to the point of pain, which could cause injury. At the point of mild muscle tension, hold the stretch for 15 to 20 seconds.

c. Breathe deeply with long intakes of breath and slow exhalations. Deep controlled breathing relaxes the muscles and brings oxygen to the muscles. This allows the muscle fibers to stretch more easily.

Types of Stretching

The stretches in this section provide the participant with opportunities to vary his/her stretching workout. When choosing which stretches to do during a session, it is important to choose at least one stretch per muscle or muscle group. A balance between agonist and antagonist muscles should be maintained. All of the stretches should be held for 15 to 20 seconds.

Achilles Stretch

This movement stretches the calf or the gastrocnemius and soleus. The person with Parkinson's stands in the shallow end of the pool facing the pool wall and grasps the wall with both hands. The right leg should be extended back at an angle with the knee straight. The left leg should be flexed at the knee, feet flat on the pool floor. The companion can help the participant establish proper balance and alignment by gently guiding him/her into position. While pressing the right heel against the pool floor or as near to it as is comfortable, the participant should lean into the pool wall. To increase the stretching effect, bend the arms at the elbows. The companion can perform the Achilles Stretch along side of the person with Parkinson's as a means of visual cueing. While holding the stretch, the companion can verbally cue the person with Parkinson's to keep the heel of the extended leg pressed to the pool floor, hold the head up and in alignment with the back. After holding the stretch for 15 to 20 seconds, the person with Parkinson's switches position and repeats the stretch with the other leg. During the switch, the companion may want to help the person with Parkinson's keep his/her balance by physically guiding him/her gently into position.

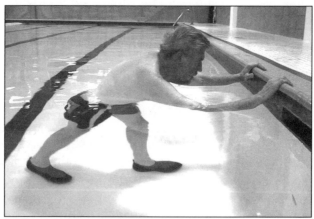

Figure 31. Achilles Stretch

Inner Thigh Stretch

This movement stretches the inner thigh or adductor muscle. For this stretch the participant remains in the shallow end of the pool with the legs spread as far apart as possible. The participant should hold onto the wall, put the bottoms of both feet against the pool wall, and lean back from the wall as shown in Figure 32. Bending the left leg slightly at the knee, shift the body weight to that leg. Then with the right leg kept straight and foot facing forward, extend the right leg out to the side. This will stretch the right inner thigh. The stretch should be held for 15 to 20 seconds and then repeated with the other leg.

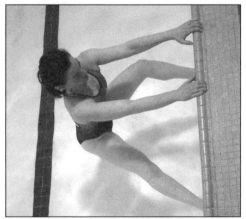

Figure 32. Inner Thigh Stretch

Should the participant have trouble balancing, s/he may want to have a partner's support. The companion should stand behind the person with Parkinson's and support him/her at the waist as shown in Figure 33. As the weight is shifted to one side or the other, the companion can help the participant keep the torso in an upright position and cue the participant to keep the knee straight over the ankle, the head up, and eyes forward.

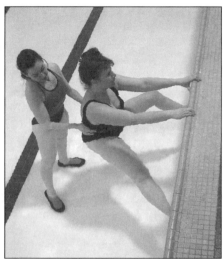

Figure 33. Inner Thigh Stretch with a partner

Hamstring Stretch #1, From the Wall

This movement to stretch the hamstring (the large muscles located at the back of the thigh) can be done several different ways. The first is for the participant to stand in either waist or chest deep water facing the pool wall. Standing at arm's length from the wall and gripping the edge with both hands, place the right foot flat against the wall somewhere below the right hand. The foot should be placed so that only mild muscle tension is felt and not any pain. For some people, this will only be a few inches from the pool floor and for others the leg may be parallel with the pool floor. Regardless of where the foot is on the wall, as long as there is a mild muscle tension, the stretch is working.

During the movement the participant must keep the back straight so that the effect of the stretch is in the leg and not in the lower back. The companion can stand behind or just off to the side of the participant and help him/her maintain his/her balance during the stretch. If the participant experiences tension in the lower back, s/he should reposition himself/herself or have a companion help him/her readjust. It is important to keep the knee as straight as possible in order to get the maximum stretch in the hamstring. As the participant is stretching, the companion can cue him/her to keep the shoulders relaxed and the head up. Once positioned correctly, the participant holds the stretch for 15 to 20 seconds, relaxes, and repeats the activity with the other leg. After completing the hamstring stretches, the participant can focus on stretching the quadriceps or the front of the thigh.

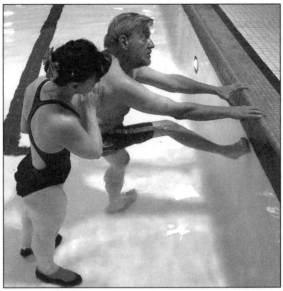

Figure 34. Hamstring Stretch from the wall

Hamstring Stretch #2

In this variation of the hamstring stretch, the participant puts his/her back against the edge of the pool. The participant places his/her right arm under the thigh of the right leg and brings the knee towards the chest. The lower leg drapes over the right arm. With the knee near the chest, the participant gently pulls the knee tighter towards the chest until s/he experiences mild muscle tension. The companion can provide support if the participant has trouble maintaining balance, and can be helpful in supporting and lifting the raised leg. See Figure 35. After holding the stretch for 15 to 20 seconds, relax and repeat with the other leg. After completing the hamstring stretches, the participant can focus on stretching the quadriceps or the front of the thigh.

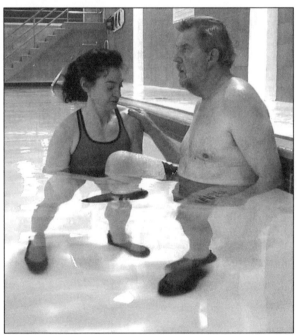

Figure 35. Hamstring Stretch with a partner

Hamstring Stretch #3, Using the Stairs

This variation of the hamstring stretch is especially good for people who have trouble with balance but do not require or want the physical assistance of a companion. The person with Parkinson's holds onto the stair rail or edge of the pool. The participant faces the pool stairs and places the right heel on a step that is at a comfortable height so that a mild muscle tension is felt in the back of the thigh. Although the companion is not physically involved with the stretch, s/he can assist the person with Parkinson's by verbally cueing him/her to keep the leg as straight as possible, the head up, and eyes forward. The companion needs to be close enough to the participant to offer physical assistance if it is needed. As with the other hamstring stretches, the participant needs to keep the back straight and arms relaxed. After holding the stretch for 15 to 20 sec, the person with Parkinson's relaxes and repeats the stretch with the other leg. After completing the hamstring stretches, the participant can focus on stretching the quadriceps or the front of the thigh.

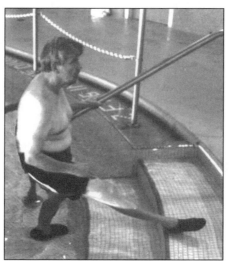

Figure 36. Hamstring Stretch using stairs

Quadriceps Stretch #1, Using Pool Wall or Stair Rail for Support

The quadriceps stretch targets the four muscles located in the front of the thigh. The participant stands in waist to chest deep water with his/her side to the pool wall, grasping the edge or using the stair railing for support. This is a good stretch for people with Parkinson's who still have substantial balance and do not require the physical assistance of a companion. A companion can still offer verbal cues related to posture as well as being close by in case the participant requires physical assistance. With knees together, bring the lower leg behind until the left ankle area can be held with the left hand. In an effort to increase the stretch, push the hip forward and try to keep the back straight. During this stretch, the knees should remain as close to touching as is comfortable and not move forward or backward in relation to each other. After holding the position 15 to 20 seconds, the participant relaxes the hold on the bent leg, returns to a normal stance and then repeats the stretch with the other leg.

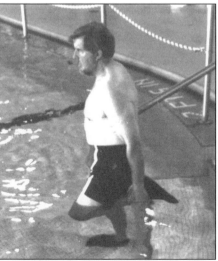

Figure 37. Quadriceps Stretch

Quadriceps Stretch #2, Working with a Partner

This variation of the Quadriceps Stretch is good for the person who has trouble with balance. Working with a partner allows the person with Parkinson's to use both hands for support on the edge of the pool wall. The companion can support the participant by holding him/her at the waist or using a hand on the participant's back as a physical guide. If the person with Parkinson's has difficulty raising the heel high enough in back, the companion can assist. The companion can help support the leg and gently pull the heel up until mild muscle tension is felt. Throughout the stretch, the companion can cue the person with Parkinson's to hold the head up and to relax the shoulders. Since the partner is physically aiding in the stretch, s/he must receive verbal assurance from the person with Parkinson's that the stretch is not uncomfortable. The companion needs to take care that s/he doesn't pull the heel up too fast or too hard. With each gentle, small increased raise, the companion should ask the participant if s/he feels any discomfort. Once the proper level of tension is reached, the stretch should be maintained for 15-20 seconds.

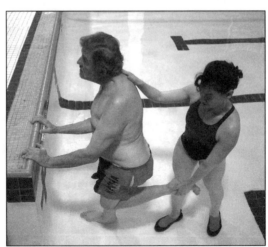

Figure 38. Quadriceps Stretch with partner

Quadriceps Stretch #3, Using the Stairs

This variation of the Quadriceps Stretch is good for people with Parkinson's who have limited flexibility in the front of the thigh. In this modification, the person with Parkinson's stands with his/her back to the stairs, facing his/her partner. Placing both hands on his/her partner's shoulders, the participant rests the top of his/her right foot on the surface of a stair at a height that provides a comfortable stretch. The partner provides added support and leverage. Instead of lifting the heel up in back, the person with Parkinson's can slowly lower himself/herself down towards the pool floor while being supported by the partner. The person with Parkinson's may also use the stair rail for balance and slowly dip down towards the floor to achieve the desired stretch while the companion looks on. This stretch should be held for 15-20 seconds. After completing the quadriceps stretches, the participant can focus on stretching the hamstring or the back of the thigh.

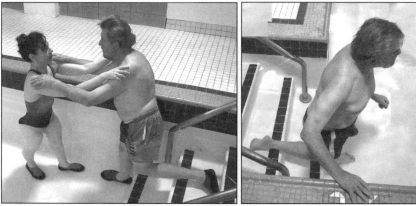

Figure 39. Quadriceps Stretch using stairs and a partner or pool edge for support

Hip Stretch

This stretch keeps the muscle that extends from the outer hip down to the inside knee supple. This muscle is called the hip flexor. If this muscle becomes short and stiff due to a sedentary lifestyle, a person will have a harder time standing up straight, causing them to have a forward lean. A stiff hip flexor also causes people to have a shuffle in their walk. This happens to a lot of people as they get older and become less active. Since people with Parkinson's are already predisposed to have problems with a forward lean in their stance and a shuffling gait to their walk, it is important to try to offset these tendencies as much as possible.

The participant stands in waist to chest deep water with the left side facing the pool wall and holds onto the edge with the left hand. Then the left foot crosses behind the right leg. With both feet resting flat on the pool floor, lean the left hip in towards the pool wall. A companion can cue the person with Parkinson's to stand up as straight as possible and to keep the head up and eyes forward. The companion can also correct the participant's form and posture if it is needed. Hold the stretch for 15 to 20 seconds, relax, and repeat the movement with the other hip.

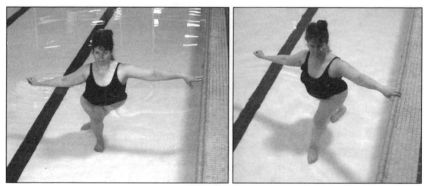

Figure 40. Hip Stretch

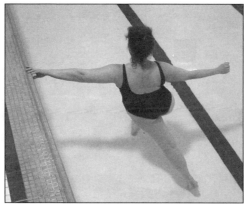

Figure 41. Hip Stretch (back view)

Side Stretch

The muscle groups affected are the sides of the torso or the internal and external obliques and the back, specifically the erector spinae. To perform this stretch the participant needs to be in chest deep water with the left side facing the pool wall and the left arm leaning on the edge. Then standing with feet wide apart, the participant reaches over his/her head without shifting the hips. This movement causes the stretch to be felt on his/her right side. A companion can help by supporting the participant around the waist and gently guiding the right arm into the proper position. After holding the stretch 15 to 20 seconds, the participant relaxes and repeats the movement on the other side.

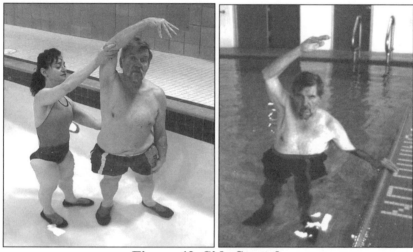

Figure 42. Side Stretch

Cross Body Shoulder Stretch

This stretch loosens up the shoulders and the back of the upper arm. Standing in waist deep water, the participant clasps the right arm anywhere below the elbow with the left hand. Take care not to grasp the elbow joint itself. Gently pull the right arm across the chest and hold the stretch for 15 to 20 seconds, relax, and repeat the movement on the opposite arm. A partner may assist by helping the person with Parkinson's keep the shoulders aligned. The companion does this by placing a hand on the shoulder as a physical reminder of where to keep the shoulder. The companion needs to make sure the participant does not twist at the waist. The companion can also help the person with Parkinson's hold the arm in the proper position by gently guiding the participant's arm across the chest. At the same time the companion can provide verbal cues to keep the head up and eyes forward.

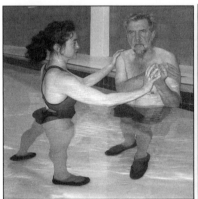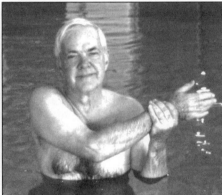

Figure 43. Cross Body Shoulder Stretch

Triceps Stretch

This movement stretches the group of muscles located at the back of the upper arm (triceps). In this stretch, the participant places his/her left hand on the pool ledge for support and raises the right arm over his/her head, bending the elbow and allowing the hand to drop behind the head. If s/he feels balanced enough, the participant can use the left hand to hold the right arm just above the elbow and gently pull the arm toward the midline of the body until there is a slight tension in the muscle. If balance is a problem, a companion can help the participant by guiding the arms into the proper position and supporting the arm just above the elbow joint as shown below. Placing the other hand along the participant's upper back can provide extra support for balance. Verbal cues include holding the head up, looking straight ahead, and keeping the body straight and upright. Hold the stretch for 15 to 20 seconds. Repeat the stretch with the left arm.

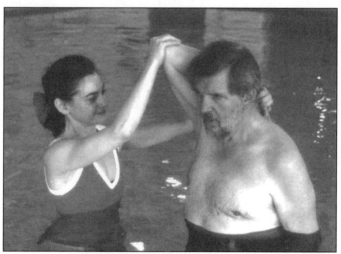

Figure 44. Triceps Stretch

Back and Arm Stretch

Stand in waist deep water facing the pool wall from arm's length away, with both hands on the edge. The feet are placed on the bottom of the pool floor at the corner where the pool wall and the pool floor meet. The participant leans backwards using the heels as pivotal points. S/he then shapes the hips, body, and head to a rounded "C" position. A companion stands behind the person with Parkinson's, placing the hands on either side of the waist and gently guides the participant into the "C" position. It is very important to verbally cue the person with Parkinson's to hold the head up. After holding the stretch for 15 to 20 seconds, the participant straightens and repeats the stretch two to three more times.

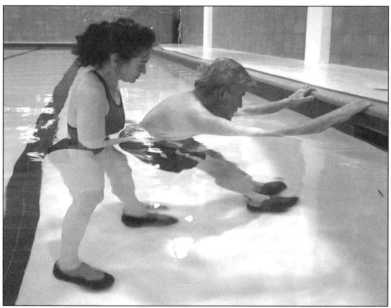

Figure 45. Back and Arm Stretch

7. The Exercises

Following the stretching activities, the person with Parkinson's is prepared to begin actual exercises. Some of the exercises involve being immersed in the pool up to chest level, while others can be done while seated on the edge. Having choices allows the person with Parkinson's to vary the exercise routines. There may be times when the person will prefer to stay mostly out of the water. Other times s/he will find the water cool and soothing and may prefer to remain in the water.

Throughout the performance of these exercises, as with stretching, it is important for the companion to give verbal and visual cues to the participant. Most of these exercises are appropriate for people who have recently been diagnosed with Parkinson's or are in the first stage of the disease. They will respond to verbal cueing. People who are in the later stages of Parkinson's will require more assistance, both verbal and visual.

Aerobic Exercises

Aerobic exercises or endurance exercises are activities that increase the heart and breathing rate of an individual for an extended period of time. Moving the large muscle groups such as the buttocks, thighs, and calves exercises those muscles as well as the heart. The person with Parkinson's should do cardiovascular workouts or other aerobic exercises that work the large muscle groups for at least 10 to 15 minutes in each exercise session.

Aerobic exercises are also called cardiovascular or cardiorespiratory exercise to reflect the fact that they increase the amount of oxygen used by the body and help to condition the heart (cardio), lungs (respiratory), and circulatory (vascular) system. During exercise the heart pumps faster and more efficiently, forcing more oxygen into the bloodstream, which improves overall health. These exercises are sometimes referred to as "endurance exercises."

Warm-up exercises can be expanded into aerobic exercises. The Water Cycle and Water Jog are excellent warm-up exercises when done for 3-5 minutes, but they become aerobic exercises when done for 10-15 minutes. Other aerobic exercises described in this chapter are The Walk, The March, The March with A Kick, The Can-Can Kick, Heel Kicks, and The Crab Walk. These exercises help improve balance and gait and are best done with a partner. It is important for the partner to be aware of the overall posture of the person with Parkinson's, especially the dropping of the chin to the chest and the forward leaning gait. If the person's chin drops or s/he starts leaning forward, cue him/her to correct his/her posture.

For people unaffected by Parkinson's disease, at least 15 minutes of continuous aerobic activity is necessary to achieve good cardiovascular conditioning. In the early stages of Parkinson's it may be appropriate to build up to 20 or more minutes of continuous aerobic exercises. However, as people reach later stages of Parkinson's they may become fatigued and 15 minutes may be too exhausting. An individual's capability and endurance will also vary from day to day.

As exercise becomes more challenging due to the progression of the disease, it may become necessary to reduce the intensity of the exercises in order to maintain the same duration. By doing so, the levels of endurance and exertion will remain the same. For example, if a person who is not in shape runs a thirteen-minute mile, the perceived intensity is the same as a person who is in better shape running an eight-minute mile. This is something the companion will need to be sensitive about when working with a person with Parkinson's.

Aerobic exercises should not be done to the point of exhaustion. The person with Parkinson's should be able to breathe easily and carry on a conversation with relative ease while engaged in aerobic activity. The person with Parkinson's and the partner need to be aware of when the cardiovascular threshold is crossed. If the person doing the exercise is too winded to speak in complete sentences, the cardiovascular threshold has been crossed and the intensity of the exercise needs to be reduced.

To vary the routine, the participant can choose to do one of the aerobic exercises for the whole time or they can do two, three, or four of the different aerobic exercises and divide the time up evenly between the exercises. If the aerobic period of the exercise session is divided up between different exercises, the companion should be sure that the transitions between the exercises are short so the aerobic benefits of the exercises are not lost.

The Walk

In waist or chest-deep water, the participant faces his/her partner who is resting his/her hands on the participant's shoulders. As the partner walks backwards, the participant follows, swinging the arms from the shoulders. At the start of the exercise, the participant steps out with the right foot and the partner moves the participant's right shoulder forward and guides the left shoulder back. While the two are walking, the partner will continue gently pushing and pulling the participant's shoulders so s/he swivels slightly at the waist.

The action of the partner guiding the person with Parkinson's helps promote a better stride and reduces the tendency to shuffle. The pair may walk from shallow to deeper water or choose to stay at a constant depth, whichever the participant finds more comfortable. Moving from shallow to deeper water while doing this exercise or any of the other exercises increases the resistance from the water. This exercise can be used as part of the aerobic workout, which usually lasts 10 to 15 minutes.

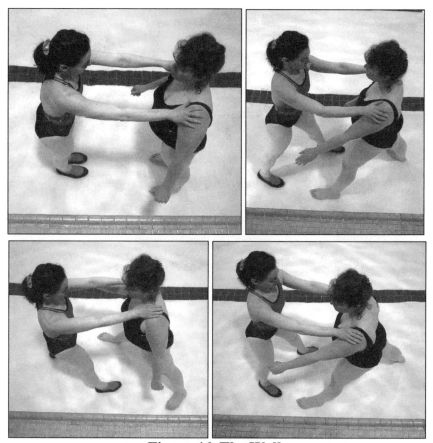

Figure 46. The Walk

The March

In waist or chest deep water with a partner facing him/her, the participant walks forward. The partner extends his/her hands forward at hip level and, while walking, the person with Parkinson's tries to make his/her knees touch the partner's extended hands. The March movement is intended to help the participant concentrate on lifting his/her feet to avoid shuffling. This exercise can be used as part of the aerobic workout, which usually lasts 10 to 15 minutes.

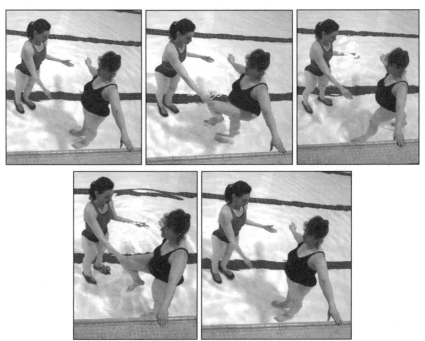

Figure 47. The March

March With a Kick

In this exercise, the partner stands beside the person with Parkinson's holding his/her forearm for support if needed. For added support, the participant holds onto the pool edge. As they move forward along the wall, the participant raises a knee to hip level and then extends the lower leg from the knee with a kicking motion. This is another exercise that promotes balance, coordination, and improves gait. After returning the extended leg to the floor, the participant raises the other knee and repeats the exercise with that leg. The partner may want to use the free hand as a target for the knees and the foot. This exercise can be used as part of the aerobic workout, which usually lasts a total of 10 to 15 minutes.

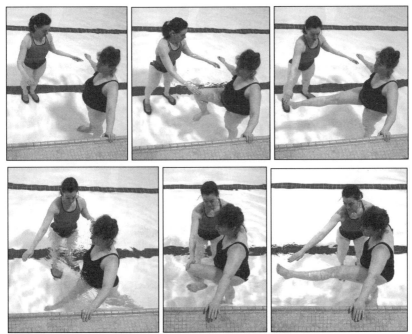

Figure 48. March With a Kick

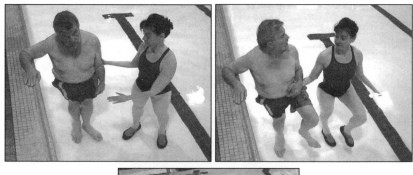

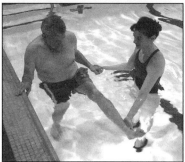

Figure 49. March with a Kick (front view)

Can-Can Kick

This exercise helps with balance and gait problems as well as aerobic conditioning. Standing erect with his/her side towards the pool wall, the participant does a leg kick, contracting the abdominal muscles and relaxing the buttock muscles during the leg lift. The action is similar to a football player making a punt or marchers doing the "goose step." At the same time, the participant swings the opposite arm forward from the shoulder with the palm facing up. S/he then alternates these leg and arm motions with enough force and speed to be challenging but not exhausting. If the person with Parkinson's feels unsteady, the arm movements can be omitted and the participant should use the pool edge for added balance as shown in Figure 50. This exercise helps promote balance since the person with Parkinson's is supporting his/her weight on one foot at a time. A companion can provide visual cueing by participating in the exercise, too. As they both proceed down the pool, the companion can offer verbal cueing such as keeping the leg straight, lifting the leg as high as possible, trying to keep the arms and legs coordinated, keeping the head up and eyes forward. Holding the participant's hand offers added support and balance as well as reassurance. If the person with Parkinson's suffers from low back pain, s/he will need to keep the kicks low. The person with Parkinson's should try to do the Can-Can Kick moving forward as far down the length of the pool as possible. This exercise can be used as part of the aerobic workout, which usually lasts 10 to 15 minutes.

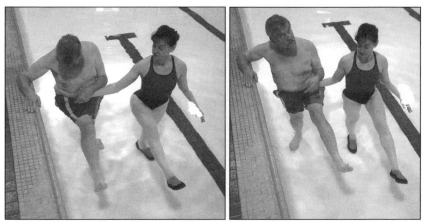

Figure 50. Can-Can Kick

Heel Kicks

Standing with the feet spread shoulder width apart and contracting the abdominal muscles, the participant stands with his/her side to the pool wall and holds onto the edge for support. Heel Kicks concentrate on the development and strengthening of the hamstring muscles. The person with Parkinson's lifts the right heel up towards the buttocks. During this movement, the person must keep the thighs perpendicular to the floor and parallel to each other. The lower leg does all the movement. The procedure is then repeated with the left leg. (See Figure 51.) This is also a balance exercise since the person with Parkinson's is shifting from one foot to the other while maintaining an upright posture. A companion can stand on the other side of the participant and perform the exercise, too. This provides the person with Parkinson's with visual cueing. At the same time the companion can verbally encourage the participant to lift the heel as high as possible and to keep the knees pointing towards the pool floor. For maximum aerobic conditioning, the participant should attempt to shift from one foot to the other with enough exertion to be aerobic. This exercise can be used as part of the aerobic workout, which usually lasts 10 to 15 minutes.

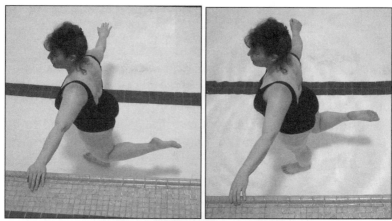

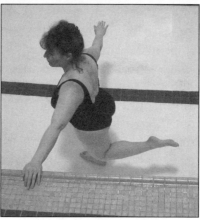

Figure 51. Heel Kicks

Crab Walk

This exercise helps develop balance and strength in the inner and outer thighs as well as aerobic fitness. The person with Parkinson's stands facing the partner in water that is waist to chest deep. Both the participant and the partner have their bodies positioned parallel to the length of the pool. The person with Parkinson's lifts his/her leg sideways and places the foot down on the pool floor. The foot is placed so that the legs are about 36" apart. The other leg is then dragged along the pool floor until the legs are together. (See Figure 52.) The participant and partner start at one end of the pool and walk sideways to the other end, and then back using the other leg as the lead leg. The cardiovascular level of the person with Parkinson's will determine how many laps can be done in the time spent on this exercise. This exercise can be used as part of the aerobic workout, which usually lasts 10 to 15 minutes.

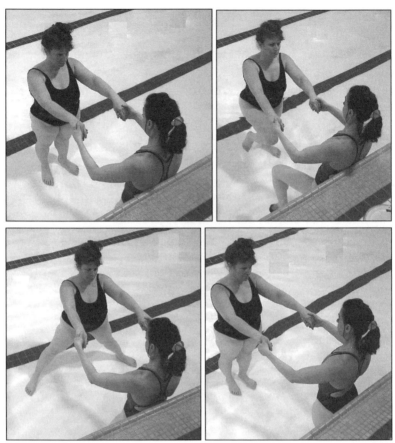

Figure 52. Crab Walk

Strength Training for the Lower Body

Strength training, resistance training, and weight lifting all refer to exercises that build muscle. Strength training exercises involve the use of long lever moves and short lever moves. Long lever moves use the entire arm or leg as a straight lever and the articulation points are at the shoulder and the hip. Since the shoulder and hip joints are ball and socket joints, long lever moves can be performed in the frontal plane, the sagittal plane, and the transverse plane. Movement can be up and down, side to side, or in rotation. Long lever moves can move in more than one plane at a time and can exercise more than one muscle group at a time

Short lever moves use just a portion of the arm or leg. The articulation points of the short lever moves are the elbow and knee, which are hinge joints. A hinge joint can move either up and down or side to side. A hinge joint works in one plane at a time and works one specific muscle or muscle pair at a time. The strength training exercises for the lower body are leg curls, knee extensions, gentle knee kicks, squats, and side leg raises. These are done in the pool in water that is between waist and chest deep.

Leg Curl

The leg curl is a short lever move done in the frontal plane and mostly strengthens the back of the thigh. The person with Parkinson's stands in waist or chest high water, facing the pool wall, and grips the edge with both hands. Standing with his/her back straight and buttocks tucked under the hips, s/he bends the right leg at the knee, keeping the front of the lower leg parallel to the pool floor, and brings the heel to the gluteus.

During the exercise the thighs of the working leg and the resting leg should remain parallel to each other. Do not allow the working leg to swing forward or backward from the hip. If the participant needs more support, a partner can stand between him/her and the pool wall and can provide support by gently holding him/her underneath the arms. Do 3 sets of 8 to 10 repetitions with each leg. Pair this exercise with the Knee Extensions to work the paired muscles of the upper leg.

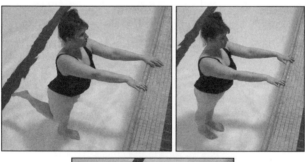

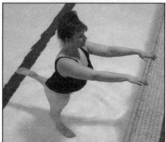

Figure 53. Leg Curl

Knee Extension

The knee extension is another short lever move done in the frontal plane and is good for strengthening the front of the thigh or the quadriceps. This exercise is done in waist or chest high water. The person with Parkinson's stands with his/her back to the pool wall and raises the right leg from the hip with the knee bent. The lower leg is then lifted up in front and outward towards the chest keeping the foot in a flexed position. Return to the bent knee position keeping the thigh parallel to the pool floor. An alternative position is for the person with Parkinson's to stand with one side facing the pool wall and resting an arm on the ledge.

The participant's partner can also help support the thigh in a raised position by allowing the person with Parkinson's to position his/her hamstring on the partner's forearm.

The Knee Extension and the Leg Curl are good strength training exercises to be done in the same workout session because the muscles being strengthened are known as paired muscles. Do 3 sets of 8 to 10 repetitions with each leg.

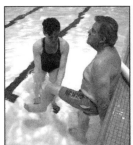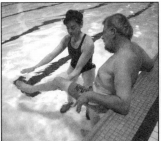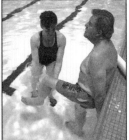

Figure 54. Knee Extension

Gentle Knee Kicks

The gentle knee kicks is an exercise that strengthens the front and the back of the thigh. This is an exercise that is done in the prone position using the pool edge, the pool stairs, a kickboard, or a noodle for support. The participant gently kicks the water by bending his/her knees. One kick with each leg is one repetition.

An enjoyable aspect of the Gentle Knee Kicks exercise is that it does not have be done as a stationary exercise. If the participant uses a kick board for support, s/he can kick down the length of the pool and do laps. When working with a partner, the partner can help support the participant by putting his/her arms under the participant's torso or can hold up the front of the kick board.

If the participant has trouble keeping the chin up, or is in the later stages of Parkinson's, this exercise can be done with the support of a noodle wrapped around the upper back. With the help of a partner, the participant lies back in a supine position and performs the exercise, as in Figure 56.

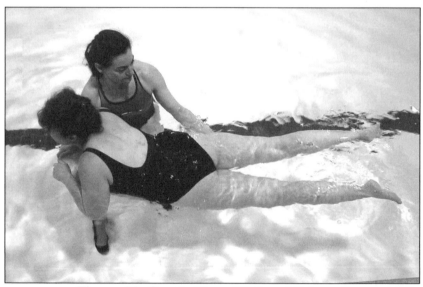

Figure 55. Gentle Knee Kicks with board

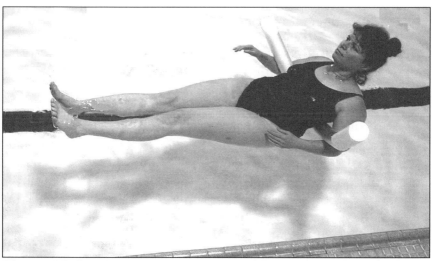

Figure 56. Gentle Knee Kicks with noodle

Straight Leg Kick

With help from the partner, the participant stretches out on the water's surface in a prone position, similar to the Gentle Knee Kicks, placing the hand on the edge of the pool. The body parts strengthened by this exercise are the hip, inner thigh, buttocks, and the back of the thigh. If using a pool that has stairs, the participant can float in a prone position and be supported by one of the upper stairs. If using a pool that does not have stairs, place both hands on the wall and grip the edge of the pool. Once supported and in position, kick the legs in an alternating fashion up and down from the hip. Be sure to keep the legs straight and kick one leg at a time. One kick from each leg equals one repetition. If the participant is working with a partner, s/he can hold the stairs or the pool edge as shown while his/her partner gently supports the torso by placing his/her arms under the participant.

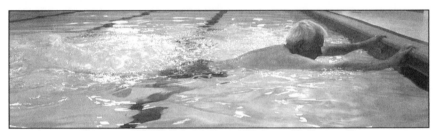

Figure 57. Straight Leg Kicks off the wall

For the person with Parkinson's in an advanced stage, the Straight Leg Kick can be done with the aid of noodle in a supine position. See Figure 58. While the partner holds a noodle, the person with Parkinson's leans back until the noodle supports his/her weight. The person lifts his/her feet off the pool floor and assumes a supine position. Once in position, the participant kicks his/her legs in an alternating fashion from the hip. One repetition is two kicks, a right and left kick. Do as many repetitions as possible in a 15 to 20 seconds interval and then rest for 15 seconds. Start with one or two sets and work toward five sets.

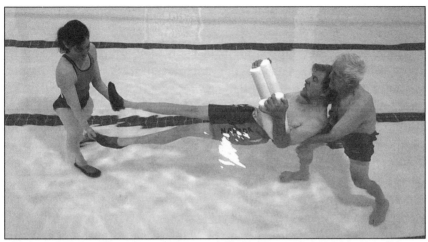

Figure 58. Straight Leg Kicks with partners in supine position

Squats

Squats work the entire upper leg and the buttocks. Standing in chest or waist deep water, the person with Parkinson's places his/her hands on the pool edge, arm's length from the wall. The participant bends at the knees as if about to sit in a chair and then straightens the knees and returns to a standing position. Feet should be flat on the pool floor and the back straight. Do not bend the knees more than 90 degrees. For more support, the person can keep one hand on his/her hip and grip the edge of the pool with the other. If the person with Parkinson's is working with a partner, the two people face each other. While the person with Parkinson's performs the exercise, the companion lends support and balance by holding the participant's hands. This exercise promotes balance for the person with Parkinson's because the body's center of gravity is shifted during the exercise. As the participant sits into the squat, the weight shifts to the heels. As s/he returns to a standing position, the weight shifts back to the entire foot. Start with 8 squats and progress to 12.

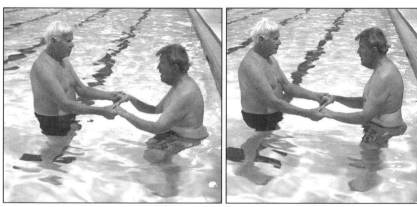

Figure 59. Squats

Side Leg Raises

The Side Leg Raise is a long lever move that strengthens the hip, the inner, outer, and back of the thigh, and the buttocks. The side leg raise works the muscles in the sagittal plane. Leaning an arm on the edge of the pool and standing with one side facing the pool wall, the person with Parkinson's lifts one leg out to the side, keeping it straight, with the toes facing forward. The participant then returns the leg to the starting position. Each time the leg is raised and lowered is equal to one repetition and ten repetitions with each leg equals one set. A partner can help by standing in back of the person, in case extra physical support is needed. A noodle or ankle weight can be used for added resistance. Do 3 sets of 8 to 10 repetitions.

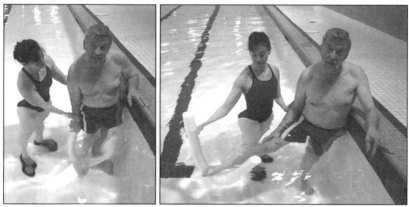

Figure 60. Side Leg Raises

Straight Leg Raises

Straight leg raises are done in waist to chest deep water and strengthen the hip, front and back of the thigh, and the buttocks. This is a long lever move that works the muscles in the frontal plane. For this exercise the person with Parkinson's stands in the same position as described for the Knee Extension. The person's back is against the pool wall and s/he slowly lifts the left leg straight up in front and then slowly brings the leg down. The foot is flexed. Lifting and lowering the leg once equals one repetition and ten repetitions equals one set. Do one set and then repeat the exercise with the other leg. A partner can offer support by standing behind the participant. Do 3 sets of 8 to 10 repetitions.

The Straight-Leg Raise can also be done with the participant standing with his/her side to the pool wall. See Figure 62. The participant rests his/her right forearm on the edge of the pool and lifts the left leg up straight in front and then slowly returns the leg back into standing position. A partner can stand off to the side to offer visual and verbal support.

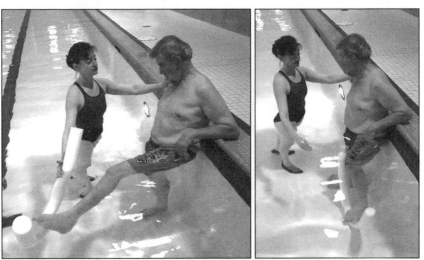

Figure 61. Straight Leg Raises

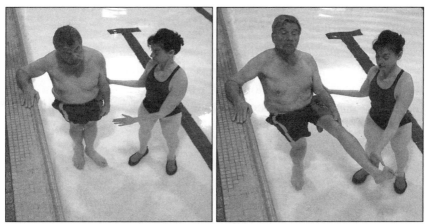

Figure 62. Straight Leg Raises holding the wall with one side

Hip Extension

The last leg strengthening exercise is the hip extension, which strengthens the hips, the hamstrings, back, and the buttocks. The hip extension is done as a long lever move in the frontal plane. The participant stands facing the pool wall, holding the edge with both hands. S/he extends the leg behind keeping the back straight and the gluteal muscles contracted. The person with Parkinson's must guard against arching the back while the leg is extended so the lower back is not hyper-extended. This will aggravate the lower back and will detract from the performance of this exercise. For added support, a partner can help by standing between the participant and the pool wall or by facing him/her and letting the participant rest one arm on the partner's shoulder and the other arm on the pool wall.

This exercise can also be done from the side of the pool wall. The person with Parkinson's stands with his/her side against the pool wall, with an arm leaning on the edge for support. Starting with the leg that is furthest from the wall, extend the leg back. When the person has completed the desired number of sets, s/he will turn the other side to the pool wall and resume the exercise with the other leg. Do 3 sets of 8 to 10 repetitions with each leg.

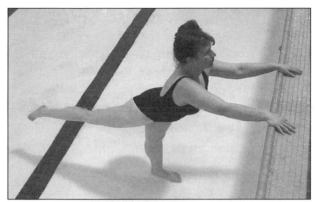

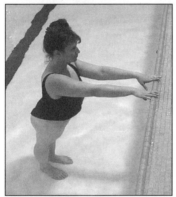

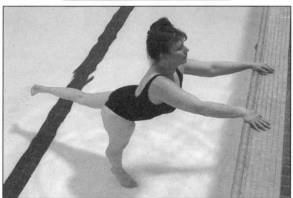

Figure 63. Hip Extension

The Side Leg Raises, Straight Leg Raises, and the Hip Extension can all be modified for the person in the advanced stages of Parkinson's. Instead of standing to perform the Side Leg Raises, Straight Leg Raises, and the Hip Extension, the person with Parkinson's can use a jogging belt which will suspend him/her off the pool floor, support his/her body weight, and keep the body in an upright position. This modification allows the participant to put the legs through a full range of motion without sacrificing correct form.

Using a jogging belt will require the person with Parkinson's to have the assistance of an instructor or partner. The partner may need to physically help support the participant as well as use visual and verbal cueing techniques to help the participant keep his/her chin up and keep the upper body steady. The partner will also need to monitor the participant's form and assess his/her level of fatigue.

Lower Body Exercises Sitting on the Edge of the Pool

Unfortunately, Parkinson's disease will progress and the person with Parkinson's will eventually find it necessary to use a wheelchair or other ambulatory aids. Despite having to use a wheelchair or walker, many of these exercises can be adapted to accommodate the needs of a person in the advanced stages of Parkinson's disease.

A person in the advanced stages of Parkinson's still needs to keep his/her muscles strong and flexible in order to stay as independent as possible for as long as possible. For people in the advanced stages of Parkinson's, these exercises build strength and endurance for the lower body in a more controlled method that is commensurate with their abilities.

The next set of exercises can be done from the edge of the pool. If the person with Parkinson's is at a facility that has a pool with zero-depth access, s/he can enter the pool using an aquatic wheelchair and perform the exercises from the chair. Other options are to sit on the pool stairs or sit on a stool in the shallow part of the pool.

Foot Circles

Although this appears to be an almost trivial type of exercise, it is amazing just how many muscles are involved. The muscles that are exercised are in the foot, the front and sides of the lower leg, and the calf. When doing this exercise, the participant sits on the edge of the pool dangling his/her legs in the water. With the right foot the person slowly makes small circles in a clockwise direction. A companion can sit next to the person with Parkinson's and perform the exercise, too. The companion can cue the participant to try to swivel the foot in a smooth, even fashion. While sitting next to the person with Parkinson's, the companion can physically cue him/her to keep the back straight and the head up and place a reassuring hand on the back. After five to eight repetitions, the participant changes direction and circles the foot in a counterclockwise direction, again for five to eight repetitions.

After completing the circles with the right foot, repeat the circling exercise with the left foot. Exercising both feet completes one set. When the participant becomes more proficient with this exercise, s/he may want to increase the number of repetitions within the same number of sets. Start with one set and increase to three sets. This will ensure the development of muscular strength.

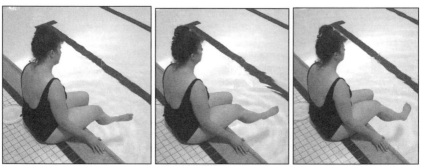

Figure 64. Foot Circles

Ankle Flexion and Extension

Another good exercise for the feet and calves is ankle flexion and extension. Sitting on the edge of the pool, with legs in the water, the participant points the toes of the right foot down toward the bottom of the pool and then extends them up toward the surface. A set for this exercise is ten times with each foot. Start with one set with each foot and work up to three sets with each foot.

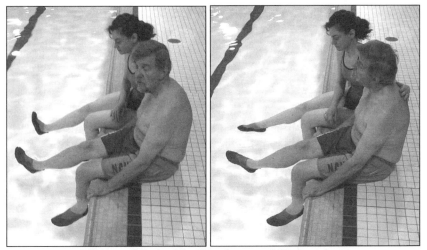

Figure 65. Ankle Flexion and Extension

The Alphabet

Sitting on the edge of the pool with legs dangling in the water, the person with Parkinson's keeps the lower leg still and forms the letters "A" through "J" with the foot moving only from the ankle joint. The muscles exercised are the calf muscles, the muscles in the front of the lower leg, and the feet. Each letter is considered a repetition and a set is the completion of all the letters "A" through "J" with both feet. "A" through "J" counts out as 1 to 10, which is easy to remember. Try to make each set more forceful. Doing a series with a different set of 10 letters of the alphabet will add variety to the workout. A companion can offer visual cueing by performing the exercise with the person with Parkinson's.

The three exercises described above strengthen the muscles of the lower legs and feet and decrease the shuffling walk that is characteristic of people with Parkinson's disease. Though part of a serious exercise routine, these exercises are fun and provide the person with positive social interaction as well as fitness.

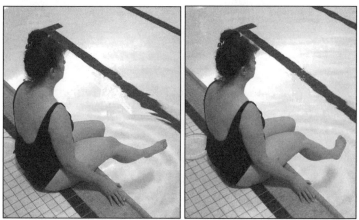

Figure 66. The Alphabet

Soccer Kicks

This is a good pool edge exercise for the lower leg, the front of the thigh (quadriceps), and to a lesser degree, the back of the thigh (hamstrings). The participant sits on the edge of the pool with his/her legs dangling in the water and with both feet flexed toward his/her body. As the participant holds the feet in the flexed position, s/he alternately kicks one leg slowly out from the knee until the foot is just below the surface of the water, returns the first leg, and then kicks the other. The flexed foot makes it more difficult to straighten the leg thus making the quadriceps work harder. Keep the feet and lower legs in the water at all times. When doing a kick, raise the foot to a point that is just below the surface of the water. See Figure 67.

A companion can provide visual cueing by performing the exercise with the person with Parkinson's. Physical cueing might include having the participant touch the top of the thigh so s/he is aware of which muscles are working. Verbal cues include keeping the back straight, the head up, and the eyes forward. One kick of each leg equals one repetition. As a precaution, keep the foot flexed to avoid strain to the ankle joint. A foot in the flexed position protects the joint and also helps to increase the resistance through the water. This helps strengthen the muscles on the front of the calf. Start with 5 to 8 kicks with each leg and gradually work up to 10 to 15 kicks with each leg.

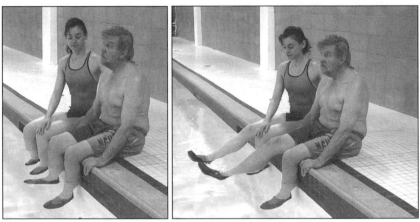

Figure 67. Soccer Kicks

Strength Training for the Upper Body

Upper body strength training involves exercises for the back, chest, arms, shoulders, neck, and abdomen. Some of these activities involve the use of gloves, paddles, or water weights. People can perform all of the upper body strength training in both early and advanced stages of Parkinson's. People in the advanced stages of Parkinson's may need to use an aquatic wheelchair, stool, or sit on the pool stairs. They might also require direct or personal assistance from an instructor or partner. The partner will likely need to help physically support the participant and offer constant cueing.

Arm Cross

The arm cross is a long lever move that is done in the frontal plane and strengthens the arms, shoulders, chest, abdominals, and upper back. This is also a good exercise to improve balance. The person with Parkinson's should stand in shoulder deep water, legs shoulder width apart, knees slightly bent, with arms straight out from the side and parallel to the surface. S/he then swings the arms down in front of the body with the hands in a cupped shape and returns them to the parallel position. The arms alternate between swinging down in front of the body and behind the back. As the arms alternate between the front of the person and the back, the resistance force of the water shifts against the person with Parkinson's forcing him/her to tighten abdominal muscles and concentrate on maintaining an upright posture. Each alternating pattern equals one repetition. Ten repetitions equal one set. Start with one set and work towards three sets. Gloves, paddles, or weights can be used to add more resistance. A companion can help by standing in front of the participant and performing the exercise while verbally encouraging the participant to perform the exercise with a full range of motion and proper posture.

It is important for the person with Parkinson's to keep the arms and hands underwater during the entire movement with the hands in a cupped position and palms turned to scoop the water so as to maximize the resistance of the water. Keep alternating between crossing the arms in front of the body and crossing the arms in back. When the arms and hands come out of the water, resistance from the water will be lost. To protect the lower back, tuck the gluteus under the pelvis.

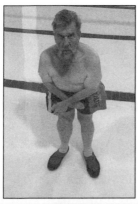

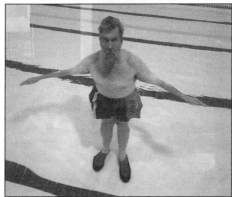

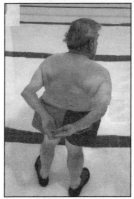

Figure 68. Arm Cross

Straight Arm Pull

Another long lever move with the arms that helps promote better balance is the Straight Arm Pull. This works the arms, shoulders, abdominals, and upper back in the sagittal plane. The participant stands in shoulder deep water with the legs shoulder width apart and the knees slightly bent. A partner stands facing the person with Parkinson's. An aquatic barbell is an ideal piece of equipment to use for this exercise. The participant holds the barbell with both hands in a prone position, shoulder width apart and parallel to each other. Starting with the arms parallel to the surface of the water in front of the chest making sure to keep the arms straight, s/he brings the barbell down towards the thighs. As the resistance force shifts, the participant's balance will be challenged. The companion will need to watch for forward or sideways leaning as the exercise is performed. If this occurs, the companion should gently help reposition the person into an upright stance. Next the barbell is lifted slowly up to the starting position. Water weights or paddles may be used to increase the resistance level of the exercise. If no exercise equipment is used, the person with Parkinson's can cup the hands. Starting with the arms outstretched and on the surface of the water, the participant cups the hands in a prone position (palms down) and brings the arms down to the thighs. S/he then turns the cupped hands over into a supine position (palms up) and, with straight arms, slowly brings the arms back to the starting position. One or two partners may assist the person with Parkinson's depending on how balanced and comfortable s/he feels. If two partners are used, one should stand in front and guide the person with Parkinson's through the exercise. The other partner can stand behind the participant and be ready to offer physical support if needed. One up and down motion equals one repetition. One set consists of 8 to 10 repetitions. Start with one set and work towards three sets.

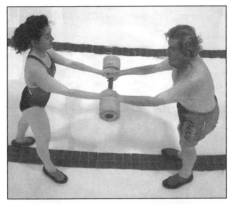

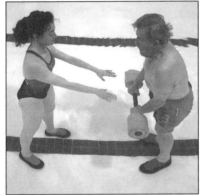

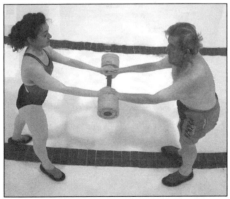

Figure 69. Straight Arm Pull

Single Arm Swing

This long lever move involves rotating the arm out to the side in the transverse plane. The participant stands facing the pool wall, arm's length away, in shoulder deep water with his/her arms parallel to the surface of the water. The participant extends one arm out and swings that arm in an arc to the side going back as far as possible while following the hand with the eyes. The person with Parkinson's then brings the arm back to the starting position. The role of the companion is to make sure the person with Parkinson's keeps the head up and follows the hand. The companion also needs to help the participant keep the chest still and facing toward the pool wall. This can be accomplished by placing a hand on the participant's back between the shoulder blades. Then the participant repeats this movement with the other side. One arc equals one repetition. Do a set of 8 to 10 repetitions on one side before switching to the other side. Start with one set on each side and progress to three sets on each side. Again, weights, paddles, or gloves may be used to increase the resistance. This exercise not only strengthens the shoulder, back, and chest, but it also strengthens the neck muscles that help keep the head from drooping.

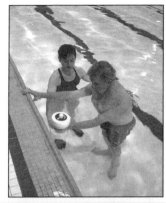

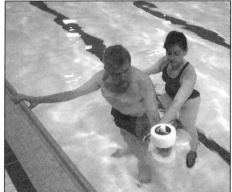

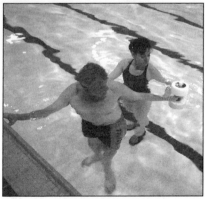

Figure 70. Single Arm Swing

Double Arm Pulls—Biceps

The Double Arm Pull is a short lever move that works the triceps and the biceps in the transverse plane. The person with Parkinson's stands in shoulder deep water, legs shoulder width apart and knees slightly bent. S/he starts with the arms fully extended, hands by the side with the palms facing forward. Keeping the elbows and upper arms still and close to the body, raise the palms upward from the elbow. S/he resists the palms as they move up as close to the shoulders as possible. A companion can stand to the side of the person with Parkinson's making sure that the upper arm is still and stable. The companion can verbally instruct the participant to keep the upper arm close to the body and can also gently touch the upper arm in order to detect any movement. Further cueing includes keeping the back straight and the head up with eyes forward. Using water weights or paddles adds greatly to the effectiveness of this exercise.

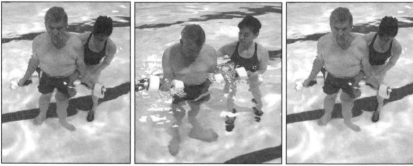

Figure 71. Double Arm Pulls—Biceps

Reversing the movement, s/he turns the hands over so the palms face down (prone) and brings the arms back to the starting position. Pulling the palms up slowly works the biceps by forcing them to work against the natural desire of the hands or water weights to float up to the surface. Using gloves, aquafins, weights, and paddles adds to the resistance. To modify this movement, the participant can extend the arms out to side, bend the arms at the elbow, and pull the palms towards the center of the body. See Figure 72. One pull up and one pull down equal one repetition. Eight to ten repetitions equals one set. Start with one set and progress to three sets. This exercise should be done with the Double Arm Pull—Triceps to balance the muscles in the upper arm.

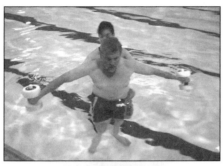

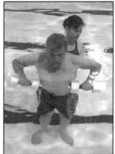

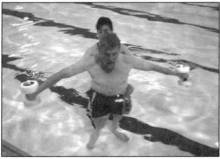

Figure 72. Bicep Side Curl

Double-Arm Pull—Triceps

This exercise strengthens the triceps or the back of the upper arm and should be done in conjunction with the Double-Arm Pull—Biceps. The set up position for this exercise is standing in shoulder deep water with the legs shoulder width apart and the knees slightly bent. The participant starts with hands close to the chest and cupped palms in a prone position (facing down). From the elbows only, s/he pulls the hands down through the water until the arms are straight. The palms are then switched to a supine position and brought back up to the surface. The companion can assist in the same manner as with the Double-Arm Pull — Biceps. This is another exercise where resistance equipment is a good addition. The double arm bicep pull and the double arm triceps pull work very well when done in an alternating pattern since they train paired muscle group. Eight to ten repetitions equals one set. Start with one set and progress to three sets.

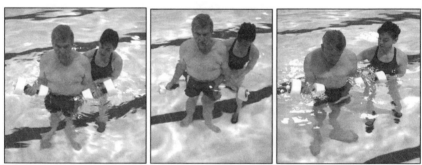

Figure 73. Double Arm Pull—Triceps

Straight Arm Raises

Straight arm raises strengthen the shoulders, back, and chest. This long lever move is done in the mid-sagittal plane. The person with Parkinson's stands in shoulder deep water with legs shoulder width apart and knees slightly bent. His/her arms should be straight at his/her side, with cupped hands and palms turned up in a supine position. Slowly lift the straight arms out to the side until they are parallel to the pool floor. Then reverse the palms so they face down (prone position) and slowly bring the arms back to the initial position. Water weights or paddles will add resistance. If the person with Parkinson's uses water resistance equipment, hold the weights or paddles with the palms placed on the top of the bar. A companion can stand just off to the side of the person with Parkinson's. One hand is placed gently on the back to help cue straight posture. The other hand is used to help the arms move straight out to the side and then back again. Each up and down motion equals one repetition. A set consists of 8 to 10 repetitions. Start with one set and work up to three.

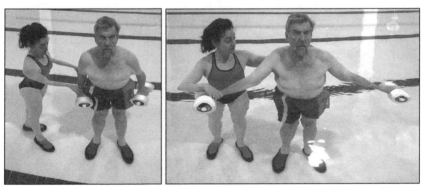

Figure 74. Straight Arm Raises from the Side

Thirty-Degree Arm Raise

The body parts strengthened are the front and back of the shoulder or the posterior and anterior deltoid. Strong shoulders will help the person with Parkinson's stand up straighter. Weak shoulders tend to droop forward and contribute to postural instability. This exercise is similar to the other arm raise exercises, only this one is done at a 30-degree angle. When lifting the arm up, the front of the shoulder is being exercised. When the arm is pulled back, the back of the shoulder is worked. As with the other shoulder exercises, stand with the feet shoulder width apart and with knees slightly bent. A companion stands in front of the person with Parkinson's and performs the exercise, too. Verbally cue the participant to keep the head up and eyes forward while lifting the arms slowly and deliberately at an angle. The companion might gently hold the participant's hands in order to help guide them in the proper performance of the exercise.

Keep the hands open and turned at an angle so the little finger slants downward and the thumb slants upward yet a small amount of water resistance is felt. Lift the straight arm at a 30 degrees angle until the arm is parallel to the pool floor then return the arm to body. Repeat. This exercise is more effective if done without resistant equipment. Shoulder muscles are not very big and can be easily damaged if too much weight is used. One up and down movement is equal to one repetition. Start with 4 to 5 repetitions and work towards 10 to 15.

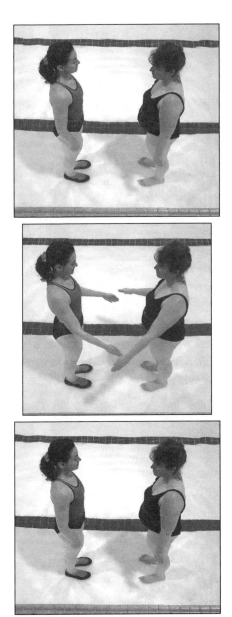

Figure 75. Thirty-Degree Arm Raise

Arm Fanning

This exercise strengthens muscles of the back, abdominals, shoulders, and chest. The muscles of the abdominals and the back help maintain stability while the arms are working making this a good balance exercise as well. The participant stands with arms straight out to the side and parallel to the floor. Keep the knees slightly bent and the feet shoulder width apart. Keep the hands turned so the thumb is towards the surface of the water and the little finger is towards the floor of the pool. Cup the hands. Bring the arms together in front of the chest with the palms of the hands facing each other, keeping the arms straight. The person then turns the cupped palms outward, reversing the position of the thumbs and little fingers and pulls the arms back into the starting position. A companion can stand in front of the person with Parkinson's and perform the exercise, too, while encouraging the participant to keep the head up and eyes forward. The partner should also watch for forward and backward leaning or listing to the side. If this is observed, the partner can verbally cue the person with Parkinson's to stand up straight while gently guiding him/her into the correct position. A second companion could stand behind the participant with a hand on the person's back for physical cueing and added support. Gloves, paddles, or free weights will add more resistance. If water resistance equipment is used, the weights or paddles should be perpendicular to the floor. Bringing the arms forward and back is one repetition. One set consists of 8 to 10 repetitions. Start with one set and progress to three.

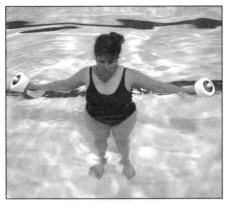

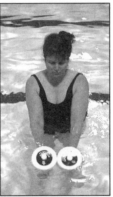

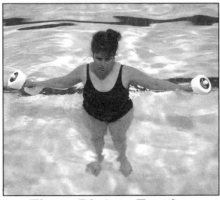

Figure 76. Arm Fanning

Straight Arm Circles

Straight arm circles strengthen the shoulders and help promote better balance. The person with Parkinson's stands in the water with the feet shoulder width apart and the knees slightly bent. Keeping the arms outstretched to the side with elbows slightly bent and palms facing forward, the participant moves the arms in a circular motion from the shoulders. Try to make large circles while still keeping the arms straight and under control.

The circles should be done so that the arms are moving backwards at the top of the circle to prevent muscle imbalance. Other upper body exercises strengthen the front part of the shoulder along with other upper body muscles. The back of the shoulder tends to be weaker than the front so it is important to strengthen the back of the shoulder in order to prevent a rounded-shoulder appearance. As the arms move in a circle, the resistance force of the water changes and the participant's balance will be challenged. A companion can stand in front of the person with

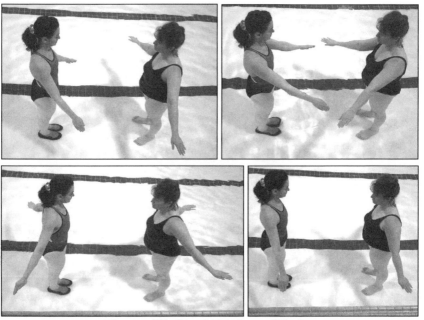

Figure 77. Straight Arm Circles

Parkinson's and perform the exercise, too, making sure the participant maintains erect posture. The only resistance equipment that might be used is gloves and only with arms held straight out from the shoulders. One set consists of 8-10 repetitions. Start with one set and work up to three.

A modification of this exercise is doing the arm circles with the elbows while the hands are on the shoulders. See Figure 78. One full circle equals one repetition. Start with 4 to 6 repetitions and work towards 10 to 12 repetitions.

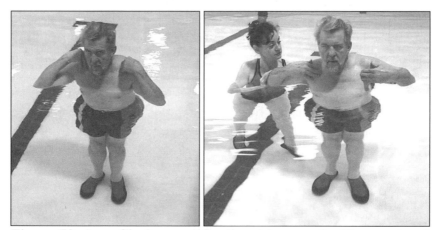

Figure 78. Arm Circles modification (alone and with a partner)

Bent Elbow Arm Swing

This is a shoulder and back strengthening exercise. Strong shoulders and backs are essential to maintain upright posture. The person with Parkinson's stands in chest deep water with his/her arm bent at the elbow at a 90-degree angle so the forearm is parallel to the pool floor and the upper arm pressed against the side of the torso. If a water weight or paddle is used, it should always be perpendicular to the pool floor. The person with Parkinson's starts with the forearm in front of the torso and swings the forearm away from the body then returns to the starting position keeping the open hand or water weight perpendicular to the pool floor. A partner may stand behind the person doing the exercise in order to assist him/her with the form as well as to offer verbal cueing. Start with the right arm and do 8-10 repetitions and then switch to the left arm. One set consists of 8-10 repetitions. Start out with one set on each side and try to work up to three sets on each side.

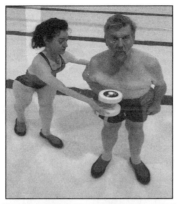

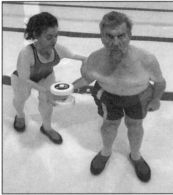

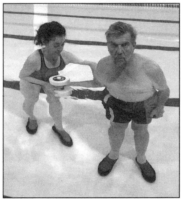

Figure 79. Bent Elbow Arm Swing

Wrist Figure Eights

This exercise strengthens the forearm and wrist. The person with Parkinson's stands in chest deep water with upper arms against the sides of the body, bending the elbow at 90 degrees. The forearm is out front, parallel to the pool floor. With the palms in a prone position facing the pool bottom and using the tip of the middle fingers as a "pen," the person with Parkinson's draws a sideways figure eight with his/her hands moving only the wrist joint. Use only the wrist and keep the forearm still. A companion can stand along side of the person with Parkinson's and perform the exercise, too, as a means of visual cueing. Another alternative is to have the companion stand just off to the side of the participant and gently hold the person's upper arms against the side. One complete figure eight pattern is one repetition. Start with 4 to 6 repetitions in a set and progress to 10 to 12 repetitions in a set. Try to work up to 3 sets. This may seem like too few repetitions but for people who have tremors and/or arthritis, this amount should be sufficient. For people who have just been diagnosed with Parkinson's, three or more sets of 10-12 repetitions may be appropriate.

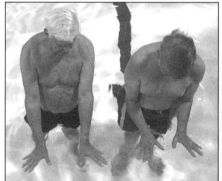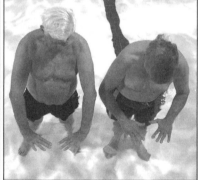

Figure 80. Wrist Figure Eights

Arm Swing with a Partner

This exercise helps to improve the participant's walking cadence by exaggerating the normal arm swing. The exercise is a long lever move and works the arms in the frontal plane. This exercise requires two noodles or two barbells. The person with Parkinson's and the partner stand face to face in waist deep water. Both the participant and his/her partner will hold the ends of two different noodles or barbells, which are parallel to each other. Both then swing their arms and, as the participant's right arm comes forward, his/her partner's left arm will swing back and vice versa. While engaged in this exercise, use resistance with each other. A participant in the more advanced stages of Parkinson's may want to sit in an aquatic wheelchair or on a stool in the shallow end of the pool. One right and left arm swing is one repetition. Start with 15-20 repetitions and work up to 40-50.

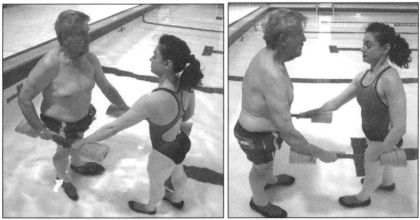

Figure 81. Arm Swing with Partner

Wall Push-ups

Wall push-ups help promote good posture by working the arms, shoulders, and upper back muscles. The person with Parkinson's stands in chest-deep water, arms length away from the pool wall and places his/her palms on the pool wall, shoulder width apart. Lean forward into the wall until the elbows bend at a right angle keeping the upper arms close to the body. Push back from the wall using the palms until the arms are straight. A partner can stand next to the person with Parkinson's and perform the Wall Push-Ups with them while making sure the participant keeps a straight, flat back. Cue the person with Parkinson's to keep the head up, the eyes forward, and the feet flat on the pool floor. Repeat 10-15 times.

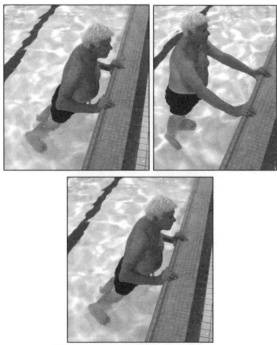

Figure 82. Wall Push-ups

Chest Press

The chest press strengthens the shoulders and the chest. Using water weights helps add resistance. The person with Parkinson's stands in chest deep water and pulls the elbows back so they are in line with the side of the body. The elbows are bent at a 90-degree angle. The forearms glide a few inches under the surface of the water and are parallel to the pool floor. If the person performing the exercise is not using water weights, the hands need to be in a flexed position so they can make use of the water resistance.

The participant pushes the arms straight out in front and then pulls from the elbows back to the starting position. A partner can help by keeping the weights in the water and monitoring form. One repetition consists of one push forward and one pull back. Start with 10 to 12 repetitions and works towards 20 to 30.

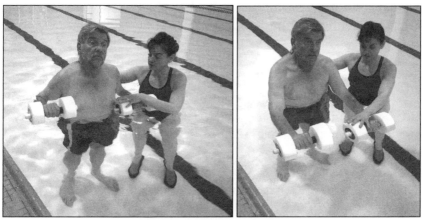

Figure 83. Chest Press

Abdominals

The next set of exercises focuses on the abdominal muscles. Abdominal muscle work is done in the frontal, sagittal, and transverse planes. When the rectus abdominal or front of the torso is being exercised, the participant is working in the frontal plane. When the participant is exercising the oblique muscles or sides of the torso, s/he is working in the sagittal or transverse plane.

Having strong abdominal muscles is very important for everyone, especially the person with Parkinson's disease. Good strong stomach muscles keep the back straight and make it easier to walk in an upright position. A weak abdomen allows the internal organs to push forward and causes a shift in the body's center of gravity. Think of a woman who is pregnant. The larger her abdomen gets and the more it protrudes, the more swayed her back becomes in order to compensate for the added weight in the front. Strong abdominal muscles help keep the body aligned and balanced.

Another issue related to abdominal muscles and a concern to a person with Parkinson's is bowel movements. As the muscles deteriorate and lose their ability to contract, it becomes harder to push the abdominal muscles voluntarily against the intestines. It is important to keep the abdominal muscles as strong as possible for as long as possible so the patient can execute private and independent control over his/her personal toilet.

Karen Bridgewater and Margie Sharpe published a study in the magazine *Physical Therapy* about the effects Parkinson's disease has on a person's trunk muscles. These muscles are located in the back, the abdominal area, and the obliques. The trunk muscles start to deteriorate in the early stages of Parkinson's disease causing gait and balance problems.

The study done by Bridgewater and Sharpe compared the trunk function of people with Parkinson's with people who do not have the disease. People with Parkinson's disease had less axial range of motion and were less able to extend the trunk region or to rotate it. The study results suggest that early intervention with a strength-training program may postpone deterioration of trunk function.

Before starting abdominal exercises it is important to become aware of how the various muscles in the abdominal area work and feel. Unlike other muscles of the body, such as arm and leg muscles, the abdominal muscles have less effective leverage points to pull against. In order to strengthen the abs, a person must tighten or contract the muscles and then work against the tightened muscles. The front abdominal muscle is called the rectus abdominis and extends from the breastbone down to the pelvis. The oblique muscles wrap around the rib cage.

When doing abdominal work it is important to breathe properly. Exhale when contracting the muscles and inhale when releasing them. Avoid arching or hyperextension of the spine during the release of a contracted muscle.

Standing Front Crunch

This exercise strengthens the rectus abdominis, the whole front of the torso. The person with Parkinson's stands in chest deep water, faces the pool wall, and assumes a neutral position with feet shoulder width apart, knees slightly bent, chest lifted, and shoulders back. The participant shortens the distance between the two ends of the front abdominal muscle by contracting the muscles. S/he brings the chest forward and the pelvis upward as if trying to meet in the center. The participant can imagine the abdominal muscles as an accordion and the chest and the pelvis are the end parts squeezing the instrument together. Another visualization that is helpful is to imagine pulling the belly button all the way back through the body and against the spinal column. A companion can stand to the side of the person with Parkinson's and perform the exercise, too, or s/he can stand perpendicular to the participant and use an extended hand to guide the person into the proper position. The companion should ask the person with Parkinson's if s/he can feel the contraction as s/he executes this exercise. One contraction equals one repetition. Start with 10 repetitions and work towards 20 repetitions.

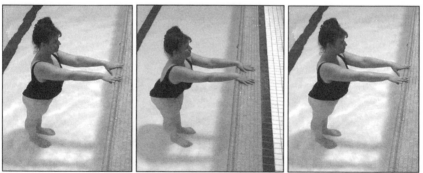

Figure 84. Standing Front Crunch

Standing Side Crunch

This exercise strengthens the oblique muscles or sides of the stomach. The person with Parkinson's stands in the neutral position with feet close together, knees slightly bent, chest lifted, and shoulders back, an arm's length away from the wall with his/her side to the wall. The participant can use the wall for balance. The person with Parkinson's makes an effort to shorten the distance between the shoulder and the hip. The hip moves to the side. Again, imagine that the oblique muscles are being squeezed like an accordion. A partner can stand off to the side of the participant and reach around to gently guide the oblique into position. The companion should ask the person with Parkinson's if s/he can feel the contraction. Make sure the participant is using the oblique muscles and is not just dipping the shoulder. Start with ten repetitions on one side then switch to the other side. Progress to 20 to 25 on each side.

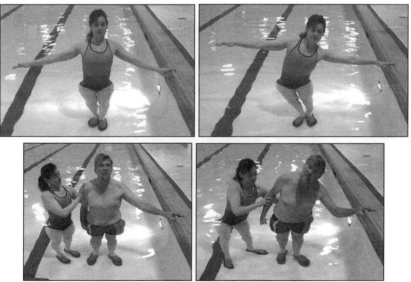

Figure 85. Standing Side Crunch

Rotation of the Trunk

This is another exercise that strengthens the oblique muscles. The person with Parkinson's stands in water that is chest deep, with his/her feet slightly apart. Clasp the hands together and extend the arms straight out in front at shoulder level. S/he swings the arms to the right and then to the left making sure the hands have contact with the water so the muscles benefit from the water's resistance. The goal is to make a 180-degree arc. A single paddle or weight can be used with this exercise. The companion may stand by to offer physical support as well as visual and verbal cueing. One arc is equal to one repetition. Start with 10 to 12 repetitions and progress to 20 to 30 repetitions.

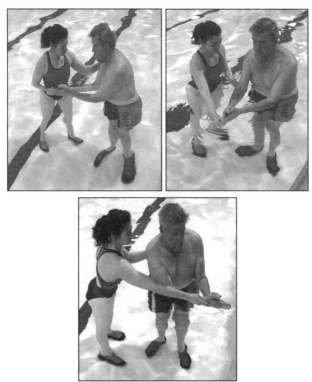

Figure 86. Rotation of the Trunk

Floating Curl

This particular abdominal exercise is the best one for the person in the more advanced stages of Parkinson's. The person with Parkinson's stretches out in the water in a supine position supported by a noodle and a partner. The person with Parkinson's has one or two noodles wrapped around the upper back and leans back while the partner stands behind or to the side and provides stabilization by holding the noodles. Extending his/her legs straight out, the person with Parkinson's trys to shorten the distance between his/her breastbone and pelvis by contracting the abdominal wall. Keep the legs relaxed. One repetition is equal to one curl. Start with 10 to 12 curls and progress towards 20 to 25 curls.

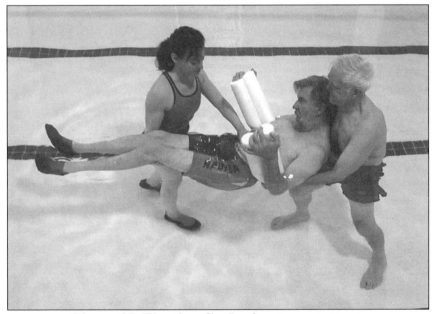

Figure 87. Floating Curl using two partners

A variation of this exercise for the oblique muscles is to try to shorten the distance between the shoulders and the hips as shown in Figure 88. The person with Parkinson's is in a supine position supported by one or more noodles wrapped around the back. The participant draws the knees up and across to the side of the chest. Then s/he straightens the legs and draws the knees up and across to the other side of the chest and returns the legs to the straightened position. Drawing the knees up once on each side is equal to one repetition. Start with 10 to 12 repetitions and progress to 18 to 20.

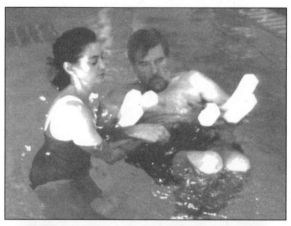

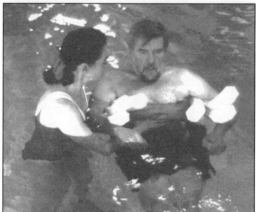

Figure 88. Floating Curl using one partner

Neck Exercises

These exercises are designed to strengthen the neck and keep the head from dropping forward. Neck exercises are performed in all three planes: frontal, transverse, and sagittal. For maximum benefit it is important for the person with Parkinson's to achieve a full range of motion. Neck exercises can be done in or out of the pool. They are good as a warm-up, cool down, or as part of the main exercise program. If the person with Parkinson's is working with a partner, the partner will need to cue the person with Parkinson's to keep the head level and straight and not wander.

Neck Extension

This neck exercise is done in the frontal plane and works the trapezius, which is located from the base of the head to the back of the shoulder blade and down to the base of the ribs. Starting with the chin on his/her chest, the person with Parkinson's lifts his/her head and looks up and back as far as possible without discomfort and then brings the chin back down to the chest. A companion can cue the person with Parkinson's to lift the head as far up as possible thus contracting the trapezius. Extend the trapezius by letting the head down. The person with Parkinson's should concentrate on lowering the head slowly and not just allowing the head to drop. The participant should do ten repetitions being careful to move the head back and forth in a slow, smooth, continuous motion.

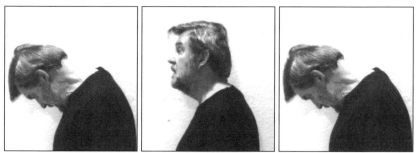

Figure 89. Neck Extension

Neck Rotation

This neck exercise is done in the transverse plane. The muscles worked in this exercise are the trapezius and the sternocleido-mastoid. The sternocleidomastoid is a muscle that reaches from the base of the skull to the clavicle or collarbone. The person with Parkinson's looks straight ahead. While keeping the head level, s/he turns his/her head, and looks over the right shoulder. The participant then brings the head back to the front and turns to look over the left shoulder. It is important to try to turn the head slowly to avoid pulling any muscles. Turn the head as far as possible while still maintaining a level of comfort. A companion can cue the person with Parkinson's by having him/her follow a hand or finger as s/he moves the head, ensuring slow, deliberate movement with the head up. Try doing ten repetitions on each side making sure the movement is level and smooth.

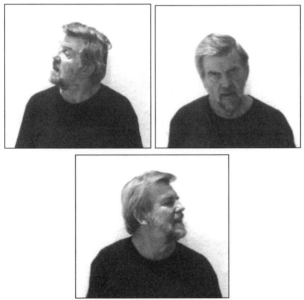

Figure 90. Neck Rotation

Lateral Neck Flexion

This last neck exercise is done in the sagittal plane. The muscles being exercised are the trapezius and sternocleidomastoid. The person with Parkinson's starts by looking straight ahead. S/he then lowers the head so the right ear is nearly touching the right shoulder. It is important to not raise the shoulder to meet the ear. The companion can place his/her hands on the shoulders of the person with Parkinson's to help keep them down. The person with Parkinson's returns his/her head to the starting position then lowers it so the left ear comes down towards the left shoulder, keeping the motion slow, smooth, and fluid. The person with Parkinson's can alternate the motion from side to side. Try to do ten repetitions on each side. The companion can watch for forward or backward leaning of the head and ensure the movement is slow and steady.

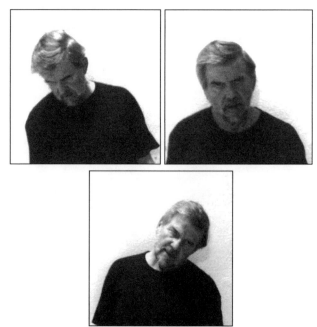

Figure 91. Lateral Neck Flexion

Cool Downs

Cool downs are stretches that are the same as those done prior to exercise, but the stretches are held for 20-30 seconds so the muscles can completely relax. It is important for the person with Parkinson's to do deep breathing during these stretches so the heart rate drops back to its resting rate. The benefits of stretching both at the beginning of a workout and at the end are an increased range of motion, improved joint mobility, improved posture, decreased risk of muscle tissue injury, improved circulation, reduced muscle tension, and a sense of physical exhilaration.

The person with Parkinson's should inhale when executing the stretch and exhale as the stretch is relaxed. As explained in the chapter on *Preparing to Exercise,* the person with Parkinson's should start with stretches for the lower body. Try to extend the stretch further after exercising than during the warm-up. However, stretching should never cause pain or discomfort. A person with Parkinson's may feel stiffer than usual on some days when s/he works out. S/he may not be able to stretch as much on another occasion. Don't be discouraged by this. The physical abilities of the person with Parkinson's will vary greatly from day to day. It is more important to stay active on a regular basis than to be concerned about daily progress.

Full Body Routines

Now that all of the warm-ups, stretches, and exercises have been described, it is time to put them together into a workable routine. Each routine should include stretching, warm-up, aerobic conditioning and/or strength training, and a cool down. The suggested programs are achievable and designed to improve and maintain functional ability. Hopefully they will promote a lifelong commitment to fitness as part of the participant's overall treatment plan.

It is possible for fitness instructors, partners, and people with

Parkinson's to design many more routines than just the few presented here. It is not necessary to do all of the stretches, warm-ups, aerobic and strength exercises, and cool downs in one session. When devising a program for the person with Parkinson's, the instructor needs to keep the selections in proportion to the body areas being trained. For example, when choosing exercises for the legs, it is important to be sure to include exercises that work both the quadriceps and the hamstrings. Do not choose exercises that work only one muscle or one muscle group to the exclusion of others. Pick out a well-rounded group of stretches so the entire body is warmed up and ready to exercise.

It is not necessary for the designer to include aerobic training and strength training in all of the routines, nor do the routines have to be designed to feature aerobics and strength training in equal amounts. Some exercise routines can be designed with a concentration on aerobic activity while other exercise routines can focus on strength training.

A good general rule for the designer of the exercise program to follow is to provide aerobic activity at least three times a week and strength training at least two times a week. How strong the person with Parkinson's feels and the stage of the disease will determine how much the person can handle.

The following pages contain some examples of exercise routines. These include many different types of full body routines such as a mix of aerobic and strength training, all aerobic, and all strength training. Common to all routines is a warm-up, stretch, and cool down section.

Some of the exercises have "balance" after them. These are exercises that are especially good for improving balance. Any exercise program should have at least one or two of the balance exercises included because this is such an important concern for the person with Parkinson's.

Included are guidelines for the duration of each section. Warm-ups routines should be done for 3 to 5 minutes, each stretch should be held for 10 to 15 seconds, and the aerobic routines should be done for anywhere from 10 to 30 minutes, depending on the physical abilities of the participant. The strength training routines are divided into sets with an even number of repetitions in each set, therefore duration will vary. To prevent overuse of the muscles and general fatigue, 15 to 20 minutes of strength training is a good guideline. If the duration of the aerobic section in a given routine is more than 20 minutes, the strength training section may have to be shortened. As mentioned before, cool downs consist of the same stretches done after the warm ups but the time for each stretch is extended to 20 to 30 seconds. The true determinate of how long or extensive a full workout is depends on the ability of the person with Parkinson's and the stage of the disease.

The number of repetitions and sets may vary. As the person with Parkinson's becomes accustomed to a certain number of repetitions, s/he may want to vary the routine for strength and endurance. There are two ways to accomplish this. One is to increase the number of repetitions per set and retain the same number of sets in a routine and the other is to retain a set number of repetitions but do more sets.

At the end of this chapter there is an example of an exercise log. See Figure 92. The person with Parkinson's will be able to chart his/her activity by noting the day, the type of exercises done, the medications being used at the time, and how s/he felt afterwards. The exercise chart will help the person with Parkinson's and those involved in the treatment keep track of progress. The log will also help determine the best time to exercise and how performance is affected by medication.

<u>ROUTINE #1. Aerobic and Strength Training</u>

Warm-up, 3 to 5 minutes
  Water Jog

Stretches, hold each stretch 10 to 15 seconds on each leg, hip, side, and shoulder
  Achilles Stretch
  Hamstring Stretch #1, #2, or #3
  Quadriceps Stretch #1, #2, or #3
  Hip Stretch
  Side Stretch
  Cross Body Shoulder Stretch

Aerobics, going lengthwise in the pool for 10 to 20 minutes
  The March (balance)

Strength Training Lower Body, 6 to 12 repetitions in each set, 1 to 3 sets each leg
  Foot Circles
  Soccer Kicks
  Leg Curls
  Side Leg Raises

Strength Training Upper Body, 6 to 12 repetitions in each set, 1 to 3 sets each arm
  Arm Cross (balance)
  Double Arm Pull, bicep
  Double Arm Pull, triceps
  Arm Fanning (balance)

Abdominals
  Floating curl, 6 to 12 repetitions

Neck
  Neck Rotation, 4 to 10 repetitions

Cool Down, hold each stretch for 15-30 seconds on each leg, hip, side, and shoulder
  Repeat Stretches

ROUTINE #2. Aerobic and Strength Training

Warm-up, 3 to 5 minutes
Water Cycle

Stretches, hold the each stretch for 10 to 15 seconds on each leg, shoulder, and side
Achilles Stretch
Inner Thigh Stretch
Hamstring Stretch #1, #2, or #3
Quadriceps Stretch #1, #2, or #3
Triceps Stretch
Side Stretch

Aerobics, going lengthwise in the pool for 10 to 20 minutes
March with a Kick (balance)

Strength Training Lower Body, 6 to 12 repetitions in each set, 1 to 3 sets each leg
Straight Leg Kick
Leg Curl
Knee Extension
Hip Extension

Strength Training Upper Body, 6 to 12 repetitions in each set, 1 to 3 sets each arm
Straight Arm Pull
Bent Elbow Arm Swing
Straight Arm Raises
Arm Swing with a Partner

Abdominals
Standing Front Crunch, 12 repetitions
Standing Side Crunch, 6 repetitions each side

Cool Down, hold each stretch for 15 to 30 seconds on each leg, side, and shoulder
Repeat Stretches

ROUTINE #3. Aerobic and Strength Training

Warm-up, 3 to 5 minutes
> Water Walk

Stretches, hold each stretch for 10 to 15 seconds on each leg, hip, side, and shoulder
> Hamstring Stretch #1, #2, or #3
> Quadriceps Stretch #1, #2, or #3
> Hip Stretch
> Side Stretch
> Cross Body Shoulder Stretch
> Triceps Stretch

Aerobics, go lengthwise in the pool with each walk for 3 to 5 minutes
> The Walk (balance)
> The March (balance)
> March with a Kick (balance)
> Crab Walk (balance)

Strength Training Lower Body, 6 to 12 repetitions each set, 1 to 3 sets each leg
> The Alphabet
> Straight Leg kick
> Gentle Knee Kicks
> Hip Extension

Strength Training Upper Body, 6 to 12 repetitions each set, 1 to 3 sets each arm
> Thirty Degree Arm Raise
> Straight Arm Circles
> Bent Elbow Arm Swing
> Arm Swing with a Partner, 30 repetitions

Abdominals
> Floating Curl, 10 to 15 repetitions

Neck
> Lateral Neck Flexion, 6 to 10 repetitions

Cool Down, hold each stretch 15 to 30 seconds on each leg, hip, side, and shoulder
    Repeat Stretches

<u>ROUTINE #4. Non-Aerobic/Strength Training</u>

Warm-up, 5 to 7 minutes
> Water Jog

Stretches, hold each stretch 10 to 15 seconds on each leg, hip, side, arm, and shoulder
> Achilles Stretch
> Hamstring Stretch #1, #2, or #3
> Quadriceps Stretch #1, #2, or #3
> Hip Stretch
> Side Stretch
> Cross Body Shoulder Stretch
> Triceps Stretch
> Back and Arm Stretch

Strength Training Lower Body, 6 to 12 repetitions in each set, 1 to 3 sets each leg
> Ankle Flexion and Extension
> Leg Curl
> Knee Extension
> Squats (balance)
> Side Leg Raises
> Straight Leg Raises
> Hip Extension

Strength Training Upper Body, 6 to 12 repetitions in each set, 1 to 3 sets each arm
> Arm Cross (balance)
> Straight Arm Pull
> Double Arm Pull—Bicep
> Double Arm Pull—Triceps
> Straight Arm Raises
> Straight Arm Circles
> Wrist Figure Eights

Abdominals 10 repetitions each
> Standing Front Crunch
> Standing Side Crunch

Floating Curl

Neck, 10 repetitions each
Neck Extension
Neck Rotation
Lateral Neck Flexion

Cool Down, hold each stretch 15-30 seconds on each leg, hip, side, shoulder, and arm
Repeat Stretches

<u>ROUTINE #5. All Aerobic</u>

Warm-up, 3 to 5 minutes
> Water Walk

Stretches, hold each stretch for 10 to 15 seconds on each leg, side, and shoulder
> Achilles Stretch
> Hamstring Stretch #1, #2, or #3
> Quadriceps Stretch #1, #2, or #3
> Inner Thigh Stretch
> Side Stretch
> Cross Body Shoulder Stretch

Aerobic, go lengthwise in the pool for 3 to 5 minutes with each walk
> The Walk (balance)
> The March (balance)
> Can-Can Kicks (balance)
> Heel Kicks (balance)
> March with a Kick (balance)
> Water Jog (from the warm-ups) (balance)
> Crab Walk (balance)

Cool Down
> Start with a Water Walk, 2 to 3 minutes
> Repeat the stretches, hold each stretch for 15 to 30 seconds
> on each leg, side, and shoulder

Exercise Log

Day	Type of Exercise	Time of Day	Medications	Results or Remarks

Figure 92. Exercise Log

177

8. Designing an Exercise Program

While it is possible for the person with Parkinson's and his/her family to design an exercise program using the information in this book, there are significant advantages to consulting with a professional for a pre-screening and a functional assessment of the person with Parkinson's. The professional can then design a program based on the findings of that assessment and on the recommendations of the patient's physician. If family members or companions, who are not fitness or medial professionals, want to design the program, they should at least have the participant's abilities assessed by a physician.

General Evaluation Tools

The most common method of evaluation is the Hoehn & Yahr stages of Parkinson's disease, which have been mentioned in Chapter 3. Other more in-depth assessment rating tools are the Unified Parkinson Disease Rating Scale (UPDRS) and The Schwab and England Activities of Daily Living Assessment.

The UPDRS is divided into three sections. The first section evaluates mental abilities, behavior, and mood changes in the participant. The second section rates the person with Parkinson's ability to perform daily activities and the third section evaluates motor skills. These areas are rated on a scale of zero to four with

179

zero being what is expected of a healthy, able-bodied person and four being total deterioration and/or disability.

The first section of the UPDRS evaluates four different areas in order to accurately assess the mental abilities, behavior changes, and mood changes of the person with Parkinson's. The four areas are intellectual impairment, thought disorder, depression, and motivation/initiative.

Section two evaluates the person with Parkinson's performance of activities of daily living. The thirteen areas evaluated are speech, salivation, swallowing, handwriting, cutting food/using utensils, dressing, personal hygiene, turning in bed/adjusting bed covers, falling, freezing when walking, walking, tremor, and sensory complaints in relation to Parkinson's.

Section three evaluates motor skills. The thirteen areas evaluated are speech, facial expression, tremor at rest, rigidity, finger taps, hand movements, rapid alternating movements of the hands, leg agility, arising from a chair using only the legs, posture, gait, postural stability, and body bradykinesia/ hypokinesia. Within the third section, tremor at rest, rigidity, finger taps, both hand evaluations, and leg agility are further evaluated to see if there are differences between the right and the left side or the upper and lower half of the body.

The Schwab and England evaluation is done by percentages. A rating of one hundred percent denotes that the person with Parkinson's can function independently. Zero percent means the person with Parkinson's is bedridden and totally dependent. The scale is broken down by percentage points with each decline of 10% representing another, more advanced level of Parkinson's disease.

The Schwab and England evaluation starts with a rating of one hundred percent, which means the person with Parkinson's can maintain total independence in all daily activities. Ninety percent is complete independence but the person with Parkinson's starts to show signs of slowness or difficulty with some daily chores. Some activities may take twice as long as normal. Eighty percent is still considered independent but chores are more difficult and do take at least twice as long to accomplish. At seventy percent, the person with Parkinson's is starting to become more dependent upon others. While still mostly independent, the person with Parkinson's takes three to four times as long to complete tasks. At sixty percent, the person with Parkinson's is even more dependent. Chores and other living tasks are done with much more effort and very slowly. Fifty percent is increased dependency. Now the person with Parkinson's is only able to accomplish half of the daily chores and has difficulty with all tasks. Forty percent is very dependent. The person with Parkinson's can do few daily tasks alone but is still able to assist others with all chores. At thirty percent the person with Parkinson's needs much more help with all tasks and can do very few unassisted. By twenty percent, the person with Parkinson's is severely disabled. S/he still may be able to slightly assist other family member with some chores but cannot perform any daily living tasks alone. By ten percent, the person with Parkinson's is totally dependent on others for everything, and at zero percent s/he has lost control of bodily functions and swallowing is very difficult. At this point the person with Parkinson's is bedridden.

More details on these scales are available on the web from the Massachusetts General Hospital's Functional and Stereotactic Neurosurgery Department at:

http://neurosurgery.mgh.harvard.edu/pdstages.htm.

Physical Evaluation

Before starting an exercise program, the person with Parkinson's should be assessed by a physician or trained fitness professional in three physical fitness areas: cardiovascular functioning, flexibility (including range of motion, posture, and walking), and strength.

Cardiovascular Functioning

To assess cardiovascular functioning (CV), a person's VO2max is measured. VO2max is the amount of oxygen a person uses when performing exhausting cardiovascular work. It is a good determinant of the circulatory system's ability to deliver oxygen to the body. Generally, the greater a person's VO2max, the better the aerobic fitness level.

Most VO2max assessment tests are done by having a person run on a treadmill until s/he has reached the point of maximum fatigue. The assessment of VO2max must be done with particular sensitivity to age and the physical ability of the person who has Parkinson's disease. It is better to use a recumbent stationary bicycle, a treadmill, or a swimming pool to assess the person with Parkinson's disease.

The recumbent bicycle is an especially good tool to use for VO2max assessment for a person with Parkinson's disease because s/he can sit in a stable position, which reduces pressure on the lower back and requires little balance. This allows the person to focus on his/her legs. Walking and swimming are also good assessment tools because the person with Parkinson's uses the muscle groups most affected by the disease.

Measuring how long it takes to run or walk five hundred yards in the pool is a good way to assess CV. One good example of a CV test was designed at Ball State University in Indiana. The test steps are as follows:

1. Calculate the number of lengths of the pool to cover 500 yards. For example, in a pool that is 25 yards long, the participant will have to cover 20 lengths of the pool.
2. Calculate the level of the water to the body so consistency in further tests can be maintained.
3. Record the start time and heart rate of the participant.
4. Have the participant run or walk 500 yards in the water as fast as possible.
5. Record the finish time and the heart rate.
6. Take time to cool down and relax.

To determine the ideal water-depth for CV, subtract 12 to 18 inches from a person's height.

Improving and maintaining cardiovascular fitness should always be part of an exercise program. For the person with Parkinson's, cardiovascular fitness information can also be used to help decide the appropriate intensity and duration of cardiovascular exercises.

Flexibility

Flexibility assessments measure a person's range of motion (ROM), posture, and gait. Knowing a person's ROM helps the fitness professional devise a program that is challenging, but not too strenuous. There are five areas that should be assessed for range of motion. They are

- Cervical flexion and extension
- Hip flexion and extension in the frontal plane
- Adduction and abduction in the sagittal planes
- Shoulder flexion and extension
- Elbow flexion in the frontal plane

Posture should be checked for any vertical deviations such as leaning forward or sideways tilt. Exercises should be devised to help correct any problems with flexibility and posture.

The last assessment is a person's gait or walking posture. The assessment looks at stride length, height of the step, and how fast steps are made. Faster steps taken close together indicate a tendency to shuffle. This is a problem because shuffling causes tripping and falling. Shuffling also indicates bradykinesia and a lack of strength and ROM. If this is a problem, the program should include some of the exercises to improve gait.

Strength

Strength assessment determines the strength of the major muscle groups of the legs and arms. Knee flexion and extension, hip flexion and extension are used to assess the strength level of the legs. Shoulder flexion and extension, elbow flexion and vertical flexion and extension assess the strength levels of the arms. Depending on the person's ability, one to ten repetitive motions should be used for this assessment. Repetitive motion refers to how many times a person can lift a certain amount of weight and what the ROM is when lifting. If the person being assessed is unaccustomed to exercise, the amount of weight used may have to be as low as one pound. The fewer repetitive motions a person can do, the less strength they have.

Exercise programs should be designed to improve strength whenever possible. Emphasis should be placed on increasing strength in ways that improve the person's ability to function in daily activities.

Program Design

Unlike programs for able-bodied clients, this exercise program needs to address the person with Parkinson's decreasing abilities rather than increasing abilities. There are other points to consider when designing an exercise program for the person with Parkinson's. The designer needs to know what physical exercises are appropriate to help the person with Parkinson's maintain balance, posture, strength, and endurance and also how to cue these exercises effectively. It is also important for the designer to understand how these exercises will translate into improved daily living activities. A person who is recently diagnosed with PD may be able to execute a program involving many stretches, warm-ups, and exercises. They may be able to participate in a full one-hour session. A person who is further along in the disease may be able to endure only twenty or thirty minutes of activity. As Parkinson's disease progresses, increased cueing may be needed and the exercise program will need to be modified and reevaluated. Frequent rest periods may be required.

When designing an exercise program for people who have Parkinson's, there are four problem areas to address: relaxation, postural maintenance, respiratory capacity, and general range of motion (ROM). Muscle rigidity makes relaxation difficult for the person with Parkinson's. The inability to relax is greatly affected by resting tremors as well. Relaxation exercises such as deep breathing and stretching are beneficial.

Muscle rigidity causes the person with Parkinson's to have forward leaning posture. This posture can cause increased back, neck, and joint pain, poor balance, and walking difficulties. These problems increase the person's chance of falling. Exercises for strengthening and stretching the leg muscles, various walking exercises, and shoulder strengthening exercises help correct and maintain proper postural alignment and decrease the possibility of falling.

Limited respiratory capacity is another result of muscle rigidity. The flexed upright position of the person with Parkinson's inhibits the muscles of the diaphragm from expanding, which leads to breathing difficulties. Exercises such as deep breathing, trunk rotation, pectoral stretching, and back extension stretching all contribute to increased flexibility of the respiratory muscles. This improves breathing ability and comfort.

It is important for the person with Parkinson's to maintain general ROM. Parkinson's disease damages muscles and joints contributing to joint adhesions and muscle atrophy. Prematurely stiffened or atrophied muscles add to the pain and immobility of Parkinson's. If a person with Parkinson's finds a joint or muscle painful to move, s/he will not move it and the problem of immobility worsens. In order to improve and maintain general ROM, people with Parkinson's should practice exercises such as trunk rotation, neck rotation, arm flexion and extension, shoulder shrugs and circles, knee extension, toe taps, and walking.

A general guideline on recommending physical activity for people with neurologic diseases such as Parkinson's was created by Drs. Charles M. Poser and Michael Ronthal. They suggest that a person with Parkinson's maintain a routine that is co-planned with friends, family, and caregivers. People with Parkinson's should be encouraged to participate in activities they enjoy but any sort of contact sport is inadvisable. According to Dr. Poser and Dr. Ronthal, swimming and other water activities are among the best kinds of exercises for people with Parkinson's.

It is possible for fitness instructors, partners, and people with Parkinson's to design many more routines than just those presented in this book. It is not necessary to do all of the stretches, warm-ups, aerobic and strength exercises, and cool downs in one session. When devising a program for the person with Parkinson's, the instructor needs to keep the selections complimentary and in proportion to the body areas being trained. For example, when choosing exercises for the legs, it is important to be sure to include exercises that work both the quadriceps and the hamstrings. Do not choose exercises that work only one muscle or one muscle group to the exclusion of others. Pick out a well-rounded group of stretches so the entire body is warmed up and ready to exercise.

It is not necessary for the designer to include aerobic training and strength training in all of the routines, nor do the routines have to be designed to feature aerobics and strength training in equal amounts. Some exercise routines can be designed with a concentration on aerobic activity while other exercise routines can focus on strength training.

A good general rule for the designer of the exercise program to follow is to provide aerobic activity at least three times a week and strength training at least two times a week. How strong the person with Parkinson's feels and the stage of the disease will determine how much the person can handle and ultimately the ideal design of the program.

9. Nutrition

Nutrition is very important for a person who has Parkinson's disease. Nutrition affects how medication is absorbed and how well it performs. A nourished and well-fueled body works better and more efficiently than a malnourished body. Having and maintaining a healthy balanced diet is essential to a productive exercise program. Knowing how nutrition affects the person with Parkinson's will help the participant, the family, and the care provider and can assist fitness professionals in designing a meaningful exercise program.

Basics

The basic principles of a healthy diet involve eating a variety of foods from the major food groups on a daily basis. These foods are vegetables, fruits, grains, meat, fish, and poultry. A principle of good nutrition is to consume less fat and more carbohydrates while watching salt intake. Maintaining a reasonable weight helps to maintain mobility. Excess weight makes moving much more difficult and that is a particular concern for people with Parkinson's disease.

Nutrients are found in carbohydrates, proteins, fats, and vitamins. Carbohydrates are sugars and starches that are found in fruits, breads, and milk products that provide the main source of energy in the diet. Proteins are made of amino acids, which help to build and repair tissue. Proteins are found in both plant and animal sources. Plants that are high in protein are nuts, grains, and legumes. Animal sources are meat, milk, cheese, fish, poultry, and eggs. Animal protein tends to be higher in fat and cholesterol than plant protein.

When there are not enough carbohydrates or fat in the diet, tissue protein found in muscles is used by the body as an energy source. This can lead to a loss of muscle mass.

Fats are an essential part of a balanced diet and are a good source of energy. Fats are found in meats, milk products, butter, and oils. However, fat is also a major factor in heart disease. Cholesterol is found in fat and is a fat-like substance that is vital for body functions in moderate quantities but too much of the wrong kind of cholesterol can lead to heart disease.

There are two kinds of cholesterol, the good and bad. The good cholesterol is HDL or high-density lipoprotein and the bad cholesterol is LDL or low-density lipoprotein. High HDL levels help the body to keep the arteries clean while a high LDL level clogs the arteries with sticky fat, which prevents adequate blood flow to and from the heart.

Vitamins and Minerals

Vitamins help the body to regulate certain processes. Most people have an adequate diet and receive an appropriate amount of vitamins. People who have an inadequate diet or who do not take in enough of the right food can develop vitamin deficiencies. There are two kinds of vitamins: fat soluble and water-soluble. Fat-soluble vitamins are A, D, E, and K. Their absorption is enhanced by dietary fat and they are stored in the body fat. Toxicity can occur when there is an accumulation of too much of fat-soluble vitamins. Water-soluble vitamins are B1, B2, B6, B12, folic acid, niacin, biotin, panothenic acid, and vitamin C. Water-soluble vitamins are not stored in the body and need to be ingested every day.

Minerals also play an important role in nutrition. Minerals are elements in the body that help to build up the body and regulate the body's functions. Minerals can be divided in to two types: major and trace. Major minerals are found in the body in amounts that exceed five grams and trace minerals are found in amounts that are less than five grams. The major minerals are calcium, chloride, phosphorus, potassium, sodium, and sulfur. Trace minerals are chromium, cobalt, copper, fluorine, iodine, iron, molybdenum, selenium, and zinc. Magnesium is considered both a major and a trace mineral.

Ideally, it is preferable to acquire all of the vitamins and minerals from food sources. However, a multivitamin can be helpful in obtaining the recommended daily allowance (RDA). A good multivitamin should have 10-12 vitamins and 10-12 minerals in the RDA amounts. Vitamin D and calcium are important for building and maintaining strong bones and teeth. Since vitamin D and calcium are found in protein and milk, people who are on a low protein diet may not get enough of these elements. If a low protein diet does not offer enough vitamin D or calcium, then a supplement should be taken.

Another very important element in nutrition is water. Water should be treated with the same importance as all the other vitamins and nutrients in the diet. The human body is 65% water. Water is important in the function of circulation, digestion, absorption of vitamins and nutrients, and elimination. Blood, which is mostly water, carries nutrients to the cells and then carries waste material from the cells. Water is necessary for temperature regulation and is the medium the body uses for chemical changes. Ideally, a person should drink 6 to 8 glasses of water a day, more if s/he is very active. Since drinks that contain caffeine act as a diuretic, they effectively reduce the amount of water intake.

Parkinson's Diet

There is a special diet for people with Parkinson's, which has resulted from the understanding that diet can interfere with the medication levodopa. Levodopa takes an hour to an hour and a half to be fully absorbed by the bloodstream and go to the brain where it becomes dopamine. Anything that delays levodopa from entering the bloodstream affects how much of the drug is able to get to the brain and how well the drug will work. Since levodopa is absorbed into the bloodstream through the small intestine, anything that delays the emptying of the stomach contents into the small intestine will decrease the amount of levodopa that is absorbed. In order to get the most out of levodopa, it should be ingested 15 to 30 minutes before meals on an empty stomach. If the person with Parkinson's feels nausea or is experiencing too much dyskinesia from taking levodopa on an empty stomach, the levodopa can be taken with a light snack such as juice and crackers. If problems persist, consult a physician.

Diets high in protein can interfere with levodopa absorption. High protein diets are rich with neutral amino acids. These acids are isoleucine, leucine, phenylalanine, tryptophan, tyrosine, and valine also known as LNAAs. These amino acids move from the small intestine to the bloodstream by attaching themselves to carrier molecules. Levodopa and LNAAs use the same carrier molecules so more LNAAs in the small intestine cause less levodopa to be absorbed and available to the brain.

The recommended daily allowance (RDA) for protein is 0.8g/kg body weight. For the person with Parkinson's it is better to divide the RDA of protein up into smaller portions and distribute the portions among several meals instead of eating the RDA of protein at one sitting. This will help reduce the chance of high amino acid levels and will increase the amount of time a person can remain mobile. Carbohydrates also play a major role in the diet because an increase in carbohydrates increases the secretion of insulin, which lowers LNAAs in the bloodstream. Therefore decreasing protein and increasing carbohydrates means that the amount of levodopa that reaches the brain is enhanced.

Herbs

Lately, our society has become more and more accepting of the use of herbs to treat various medical conditions including Parkinson's disease. The use of herbs as medicine is not new and dates back thousands of years. Herbs are plants that have medicinal qualities due to their chemical composition, making them useful as drugs. Many of our modern prescription drugs are made from herbs. The problem with using herbs as medicine is that they are not regulated by government agencies. Since herbs are not regulated, the amount of herbs to be used, or that are contained in herbal products is uncertain. Furthermore, there are no quality standards that are established and enforced. The information that exists on the effectiveness and safety of herbs is limited and is often not based on sound scientific research or testing. In 1994 the U.S. Congress passed a law called the Dietary Supplement Health and Education Act or DSHEA. According to the DSHEA, herbs produced as dietary supplements are considered to be safe unless proven otherwise. The herbal-as-medicine market has grown because such herbs and their claims are not subjected to clinical trials and tests as are pharmaceuticals. Manufacturers of herbal medicines are not required to disclose or record complaints by consumers.

Many people are persuaded to try herbs as an alternative to conventional medication and/or vitamin supplements because herbs are advertised as "natural" remedies. This implies that conventional diets and medications are unnatural. People also assume that the phrase "all natural" is synonymous with "no side effects" which is far from true. This type of thinking plays upon people's fear of ingesting harmful chemicals. As mentioned before, many medications and vitamin supplements come from natural products. For example, aspirin comes from the willow bark. It is much easier however, to take aspirin in its refined state as a pill rather than to chew on a piece of bark.

Natural also does not necessarily mean that a product is good for you. Hemlock is a natural herb with deadly effects. There are other negative consequences of using herbs. By using herbs as an alternative, serious health problems could be neglected or the use of more effective medical treatment may be ignored or delayed. Overuse of herbs could prove to be toxic, especially when the amount to be used safely is not known. Herbs may also interfere with an ongoing medication program.

As of now, little is known about how herbs affect the primary symptoms of Parkinson's. Herbs can be beneficial and safe if used under the supervision of a trained medical professional. It is possible that certain herbs can be used to help treat problems occurring due to a Parkinson's symptom or a medication side effect. Conditions related to Parkinson's that may benefit from herbal remedies are constipation, nausea, indigestion, depression, pain, sleep disturbance, cognitive changes, anxiety, and urinary problems in men.

People with Parkinson's who suffer from constipation can be helped with the widely used herb senna, which is inexpensive and quite safe. An even milder herb for relieving constipation is cascara. Nausea can be treated with the herb ginger. However if the person with Parkinson's is taking an anticoagulant, ginger should be avoided because it can prolong bleeding time. Peppermint in the form of a mild tea can help indigestion, but too much can be toxic. Chamomile tea is also used for indigestion. Chamomile can be helpful with inflammation and with gum irritation. People who are allergic to Asteraceae, ragweed, chrysanthemums, or asters should avoid chamomile.

St. John's wort has ingredients called flavonoids, hypericin, and xanthenes which may help with the symptoms of mild to moderate depression. It should not be used with other anti-depressants. Severe depression requires medical treatment. If a person with Parkinson's uses St. John's wort, s/he should avoid exposure to the sun.

Applying a topical mixture of mineral oil and cayenne pepper to an affected area can temporarily relieve muscle or joint pain. Since cayenne is a strong irritant, eye contact should be avoided and the hands should be thoroughly washed afterwards.

Sleep disturbance and anxiety can both be treated with valerian root. Valerian root appears to reduce nervous tension, restlessness, and stress without being addictive or impairing motor functions. Since valerian root may help reduce nervous tension, sleep quality may improve. However, valerian root can decrease blood pressure. If a person with Parkinson's is on blood pressure medication, s/he should speak to his/her doctor before taking valerian root. Valerian root should not be mixed with alcohol.

Cognitive changes may be helped by gingko biloba. Gingko biloba contains the antioxidant flavonoid and terpene lactones, which may help with concentration, memory, confusion, depression, tinnitus, headaches, vertigo, and peripheral circulation. Gingko biloba may also help alleviate Sinemet's side effect of daytime sleepiness. The negative effects of gingko biloba are an increase in blood glucose levels and prolonged bleed time in people with bleeding disorders.

Huperzine A is a Chinese herbal extract that helps to restore the neurotransmitter acetylcholine. Huperzine A is stronger than gingko biloba.

The herb saw palmetto may help men with urinary problems by reducing the size of the prostrate gland which leads to decreased frequency of urination, reduced residual urine, and increased urinary flow. Before taking saw palmetto for urinary problems, prostate cancer or other causes of the symptoms need to be ruled out by a physician.

The five most harmful herbs are chaparral, comfrey, ephedra, lobelia, and yohimbine. All of these herbs have supporters that claim they will perform medical miracles. These "miracles" have not been substantiated, but these herbs have documented, serious side effects.

Chaparral is a natural antioxidant, which is promoted as a blood purifier that can cure ailments from acne to cancer. Chaparral has been implicated in six cases of acute nonviral hepatitis. In one case, a patient required a liver transplant. Chaparral is sold as a single herb or it can be found as an ingredient in herbal formulas. Check the ingredients of any "natural" products before buying them.

Comfrey, like chaparral, is promoted as a blood purifier as well as a tonic to reduce pain from arthritis. Comfrey also contains alkaloids that are toxic to the liver. Comfrey has been implicated in seven cases of food obstruction due to reduced liver function. Such obstruction causes scarring of the liver (cirrhosis).

Ephedra is more commonly known as ephedrine and can be found in herbal products like ma luang, Chinese ephedra, and Sida cordifloia. Ephedra claims that it promotes weight loss and enhances athletic abilities. Ephedra is a decongestant and stimulant similar to amphetamines. Ephedra can help relieve bronchial asthma but the side effects include increased heart rate and blood pressure. Since ephedra is a stimulant, using it with other stimulants such as caffeine, can intensify ephedra's adverse side effects. Since 1993, the FDA has reported that 17 people have died and 800 have been become seriously ill by using products containing ephedra.

Yohimbine claims to increase muscle mass, reduce body fat, and act as an aphrodisiac. None of these claims has been substantiated. The FDA has proclaimed yohimbine to be ineffective for its intended use and generally unsafe. An overdose of yohimbine can cause nervous stimulation and weakness. It has been known to cause paralysis, fatigue, stomach disorders and even death. Yohimbine reacts negatively with foods such as red wine, liver, and cheese because they contain tyramine. Yohimbine can cause hypertensive reactions if taken in conjunction with decongestants or foods containing phenylpropanolamines. People who suffer from heart, liver, or kidney disease, or have diabetes or hypertension should not use yohimbine. Anyone who uses this herb should do so under the care of a physician.

Lobelia is reputed to have antispasmodic effects and is used to enhance respiratory function. It also claims to suppress the desire for nicotine. Native Americans called lobelia "pukeweed" because if a person ingested too much, s/he would become nauseated and vomit. Lobelia is toxic and signs of lobelia poisoning are heartburn, weak pulse, troubled breathing, and general fatigue.

10. Frequently Asked Questions

This section discusses questions that are frequently asked by people with Parkinson's disease. Tom Mraz, a client and friend of mine who is living with Parkinson's disease, submitted many of the questions to me concerning water exercise. I asked Tom to generate questions because I felt he had an intimate understanding of what people with Parkinson's really want to know.

1. I have just been diagnosed with PD. When should I start an exercise program?

Since Parkinson's disease is progressive, a person who has just found out that s/he has PD should start an exercise program as soon as possible. The symptoms of Parkinson's get worse over time and they also become more numerous. Exercise will help delay the progression of the disease and give the newly diagnosed person with Parkinson's a chance at a more independent life for a longer period of time. The worst response to the diagnosis of Parkinson's is to do nothing. Inactivity will lead to muscle atrophy, which will allow the disease to progress at a faster pace.

2. Why should I do water exercises?

The properties of water are such that there is less stress on the joints. The water offers continuous yet gentle resistance. The water keeps the body cooler so the person with Parkinson's doesn't fatigue as quickly due to excess body heat. Since a person is buoyant in the water, balance is easier to maintain. Water exercises, as with any exercise, helps to alleviate isolation, depression, and anxiety.

Among the physiological benefits of water exercise are improved circulation, mobility, strength, coordination, range of motion, pulmonary function, perceptual and spatial awareness, muscular and cardiovascular endurance, relaxation, and increased bone mass. The psychological benefits are enhanced mood, self-esteem, and body image. Physical activity for people with Parkinson's helps the person remain physically independent for a longer period of time. However, a person with Parkinson's should consult with his/her physician and have his/her physical abilities assessed by a fitness professional or physical therapist before embarking on an exercise program.

3. Is exercising in the water a good and valuable method of helping the person with Parkinson's?

Yes. Exercising in the water is fun and an effective way to improve stride, strength, flexibility, range of motion, and muscle tone without putting stress on joints, bones, and muscles. Water provides a perfect medium for working on the cardiovascular system. Exercising in the water is also an effective way to engage in balance and resistance training, which is important in maintaining an upright, steady walk and preventing falling.

In one study conducted by Marjorie Johnston, Clinical Exercise Specialist for the Southwest Florida Parkinson's Association, eleven people aged 63-88 in different stages of Parkinson's engaged in one hour of water exercise three times a week from the period of January through May 2000. Before participating in the water exercise program, the participants were given assessment tests for strength, flexibility, balance, and mobility. The people in the study performed water exercises that targeted walking, gait, balance, strength, and flexibility. Water equipment such as gloves, paddles, noodles, and aquatic steps were used to aid the participants. At the end of the study, the participants were reassessed. Four of the eleven improved in all of the areas tested, three improved in the majority of the areas tested, and the other four improved in half of the areas tested. All of the people had improved levels of function. Some also experienced reduced feelings of depression, a reduction of their medication, less pain, and reduced muscle rigidity.

In another study, done by M. A. Hirsch at Florida State University, the effects of balance and resistance training were tested. Participants were put into two groups. One group received balance and resistance training while the other group received only balance training. In the group that received both balance and resistance training, muscle strength increased and incidents of falling were reduced. In the group that received only balance training, muscle strength was not substantially improved. The study concluded that people with Parkinson's disease benefit greatly from a combination of balance and resistance training.

The two studies combined to show that water exercise helps a person with Parkinson's regain physical abilities that lead to a fuller, more independent lifestyle. It is worthwhile to participate regularly in water exercise.

4. Are doctors able to use water exercises as a treatment for Parkinson's disease?

Water exercises can be incorporated as part of an overall treatment program that includes diet, medication, and possibly surgery. Many doctors advocate exercise as part of a treatment plan for people with Parkinson's. Exercising in the water is just one of many choices when deciding what physical activity is best.

The symptoms of Parkinson's can be improved by many different kinds of exercise including water exercises. Research has shown that exercise affects both direct and indirect symptoms of Parkinson's disease. The direct symptoms are tremor, bradykinesia, rigidity, and imbalance. The indirect symptoms are loss of muscle strength, range of motion, and cardiorespiratory function. With exercise, the direct symptoms are reduced and the indirect symptoms are improved.

Dr. James Tetrud, M.D., a member of the Board of Directors at the Parkinson's Institute in Sunnyvale, CA says, "Exercise for individuals with Parkinson's disease is much more than a pursuit of physical fitness. It is a lifelong necessity and as much a part of the treatment program as the medication."

5. Does working out in a pool make you more susceptible to infections?

Pool water is treated chemically to prevent bacterial growth. The pool water is also filtered continuously for safety and comfort. The real key to keeping the body free from infection is to dry off properly after each workout. If a person is susceptible to fungus outbreaks, dry these areas thoroughly and use a powder or cream that is made for these conditions.

Before getting into a pool, check the odor, clarity, and cleanliness of the water. If there is a chronic "ring around the collar" then look for another pool. Women don't need to worry about water entering the vagina. The position of the anterior and posterior walls keeps the genitals protected.

6. Is chlorine harmful?

Chlorine is a chemical used in pools to keep them free of bacteria and algae. It is not harmful but can dry the skin and hair. In rare occasions, it will irritate the eyes even if a person does not submerge his/her head in the water. If that is the case, try wearing goggles. If the skin feels dry and itchy after being in the pool, apply moisturizer to the skin.

7. Do I need to protect my ears?

All of the exercises in this book are done with the head out of the water. However if a person wishes to prevent water from splashing into the ear canal, s/he can wear earplugs, a swim cap, or apply lamb's wool to the outer ear canal and seal it with petroleum jelly.

8. In what ways are the water exercises going to help people with Parkinson's?

Water exercises will help improve balance, coordination, muscle tone, muscle strength, and muscle flexibility. Water exercise will also help the person with Parkinson's walk with a better stride. Since the buoyancy factor of the water helps to support the person with Parkinson's, s/he will take longer strides while walking in the water. S/he will continue this practice when walking on land.

A study was done in the United Kingdom and Germany to assess the value of therapeutic exercise training for people with Parkinson's. The study was conducted over a 20-week period and involved 16 people with idiopathic Parkinson's disease. The program consisted of sessions in warm water and in a gymnasium. After the program was over, the results gathered from the progress of the participants showed that an intensive exercise program improves motor function as well as an overall feeling of well being.

9. Will water exercises be any help for my worsening posture?

Yes. When a person stands in the pool, the water exerts pressure on the body from all sides. As mentioned in Chapter 1, this hydrostatic pressure forces the core stabilizers (the muscles in the torso) to contract and tighten against the water's pressure. Hydrostatic pressure causes the person to stand in an upright position. The muscles in the abdomen and the back make up the torso area. The resisting force of the water helps to promote balance by providing resistance to movement in all directions. Working and strengthening the core stabilizers in the torso helps the person with Parkinson's to stand more upright.

In the study mentioned in the previous answer, the training session that focused on resistance training and reducing trunk rigidity took place in water. Walking with a firmer, longer, surer stride shifts the center of gravity in the body and makes it easier to walk more upright. Working against the resistance of the water helps to strengthen the muscles. Buoyancy provides a cushioning effect. Stooped posture can also be helped by looking straight ahead and not down at one's feet. Keeping the shoulders, chest, upper back, and neck muscles strong will help make it easier to hold a better posture.

10. How will water exercise help my slurred speech?

Reduced movement of the muscles that control breathing and the vocal chords causes problems related to speech. Consequently the ability to articulate and the rhythm, intonation, and rate of speaking are affected. All of these muscles are found in the face, head, neck, and the diaphragm. The best therapy for speech dysfunction is to do facial exercises and engage in speech therapy.

The muscle that water exercise will help is the diaphragm. A strong diaphragm is a major part of speaking ability. Exercise forces a person to breathe deeply and regularly. Regular deep breathing increases the oxygen levels in the muscles and helps them to work more efficiently. While exercising with a partner, the person with Parkinson's should engage in conversation using speech therapy techniques such as exaggerated facial expression, speaking in short concise sentences, and concentrating on enunciating the words.

11. Will water exercises help my self-confidence?

YES! Being with people while exercising and social interaction will make the person with Parkinson's feel better about himself/herself. Also, the improvement of posture, gait, strength, and flexibility will give him/her more confidence. The more a person is able to prove that s/he can lead an active, independent life, the better s/he will feel. Exercising not only improves a person's physical abilities, but also helps to boost a person's self-esteem and improves his/her emotional state of mind.

12. Do I have enough strength to do exercises in the water?

This answer depends on the intensity of the exercise and the stage of the disease. Generally, if a person has the strength to walk and move about, s/he will have enough strength to do simple exercises. As the disease progresses, modifications and variations can be made to make the exercises more manageable. Doctors and other caregivers rate swimming and water activities among the best exercises for people with Parkinson's.

13. Am I strong enough to swim in the pool?

Once a person with Parkinson's has been assessed by a professional caregiver and assuming s/he can walk and move about, s/he can swim. There are many levels of swimming. Some people will use a kick board for support and be propelled by their legs, or they may swim using both arms and legs but only do one lap. Swimming means different things to different people. One does not need to be an Olympic athlete to enjoy a good swim.

14. Am I strong enough to swim or engage in water exercises alone?

One of the many fears people with debilitating diseases have is losing their independence. People with healthy bodies take for granted that they can go anywhere and do anything on their own without having someone watching over them. Unfortunately, people with Parkinson's suffer from a condition known as freezing. If this happens while a person is in the water, s/he could drown because muscles bind or freeze. Also, people with Parkinson's can become fatigued suddenly and may require assistance to exit the pool. For the person with Parkinson's, it is important for safety reasons and for the family's peace of mind, to either swim with a companion or to go to a facility where there is a lifeguard who is familiar with Parkinson's.

The friends and family of the participant need to appreciate the person's desire for solitude and privacy. That means being aware of where the person with Parkinson's is but not hovering over him/her, or falling into the trap of treating the person as an infant, or speaking about the participant in the third person while in his/her presence.

15. Will water exercises take too much of my strength to be beneficial?

Almost half of the people who have Parkinson's suffer from fatigue and have a tendency to remain inactive. Being inactive leads to muscle atrophy, which leads to even less energy and activity. It is a vicious circle. Fears that fatigue from exercise will cause physical setbacks are unfounded. Despite the fact that a person has Parkinson's, it is important to remain as active as possible. If a person with Parkinson's works at the recommended intensity for his/her condition, then water exercises will not be too strenuous. Since water keeps the core body temperature lower, it takes longer to get fatigued. Water also provides gentle but constant weight resistance.

16. What can I do when I freeze up?

When exercising, a person with Parkinson's may feel that one foot seems to stick to the pool floor, becoming immobile or frozen. This phenomenon may or may not occur frequently and usually occurs in doorways, during turns, and while crossing streets or walkways. In order to become unfrozen the person with Parkinson's should remain calm and try to concentrate on lifting the toes and visualize stepping over an object in front of his/her path. S/he should place the heel of the foot on the ground, tap the hip of the leg that s/he wants to move, or try to march in place.

17. What should I do if I feel any discomfort?

If there is any feeling of physical discomfort then the person with Parkinson's should stop and rest. If the discomfort goes away in a few minutes, try to continue. If the discomfort persists, then the body is trying to signal that something is not right and a visit to a physician may be appropriate.

18. Are there age limitations to when someone can start an exercise program?

A person is never too old to start an exercise program. Studies have shown that people in their eighties and nineties have cardiovascular and muscular improvement after being put on an exercise program. For some, it has meant the difference between getting out of a chair on their own or waiting for assistance. In one study, people age 80 and older participated in a ten-week strength-training program and progressed from using walkers to using canes.

Regular exercise benefits older adults and people with disabilities. People tend to become sick or disabled much more often from a lack of exercise than from participating in exercise. People with disabilities improve both physically and mentally with regular exercise. It is wise to get a physical examination before starting an exercise program. If a person has not exercised before, water exercise is the best all-around activity because it is not as strenuous or jarring to the joints and bones as land activities.

19. Will my muscles feel sore after my workout and what should I do about it?

A person may feel sore after working out, especially if just starting an exercise program. Muscles get sore if they have not been active for a while. Be sure to warm up and stretch before each workout. Start workouts slowly at first and try to follow a program for three times a week. After each workout be sure to cool down and stretch so the muscles can relax. As exercise increases, soreness will decrease. With consistent exercise, the muscles become more responsive to the demands placed upon them. If pain or discomfort persists, consult with a physician.

20. Should I drink anything after my workout?

YES! Water. Drink water before, during, and after each workout. It is important to be hydrated before working out so there is less stress on the circulatory system. Exercise uses up the water supply and people become dehydrated even if they do not feel thirsty. Even though working out in the water may not leave a person sweaty, s/he will perspire and need to replenish his/her water supply. Drinking cool water, not ice cold, is best. Cool water enters the bloodstream at a faster rate than ice cold.

If a person feels thirsty, s/he is already dehydrated. Try to drink sixty-four ounces of water a day. Monitor the hydration level by looking at the color of the urine. The urine should be a pale yellow. If it is darker, then the person is not getting enough water.

21. What should I do if I become discouraged about my program?

First of all, DON'T GIVE UP! There are no short cuts to physical fitness. It takes persistence, dedication, and self-discipline. It is not unusual to be discouraged. It is important to remember that exercise will promote the development of a healthy, happier, more independent person. Savor the success of walking a little farther or being able to do an activity unassisted. With dedication, the discouragement will pass.

Above all, have a positive attitude. According to the U.S. Surgeon General, a person is likely to stick with an exercise program if s/he thinks from the start that s/he will succeed. To achieve success, set realistic goals, learn to perform the exercises correctly, and chart the progress so improvement can be seen. Celebrate achieving realistic goals with great regularity.

Sid Dorros, a person living with Parkinson's, devised a strategy to help participants prevent discouragement. He calls the strategy the Three R's: Reason, Regularity, and Reality. An activity that has reason or purpose or is enjoyable will be easier to follow on a regular basis versus a dull and unenjoyable activity. Doing an activity that is enjoyable at a regular time on certain days will help the activity become part of an established routine. A person with PD must be realistic about his/her physical abilities. It is important to set realistic goals and take a realistic approach to achieving them. If a person can stick to a program for more than a month, it is a good sign that exercising will become part of a routine or life style.

22. I am very busy, how can I find time to exercise?

Establish an exercise program as a high priority activity. It pays great dividends, especially for the person with Parkinson's. Try to schedule at least one hour or more for exercise and all that it includes, three days a week, without fail. People deserve that much time for themselves. Treating exercise with the same importance as a job may help establish exercise as a regular part of the treatment routine. The person with Parkinson's needs to discuss his/her desire to exercise with family, friends, and a physician. Once family and friends understand that the person with Parkinson's is serious, they will probably support the efforts and may even become involved in exercising, too.

23. Should I use water equipment right away?

Before a person with Parkinson's attempts to use water equipment, his/her strength and abilities need to be assessed by a therapist, fitness trainer, physician, or qualified companion. If the person is in the habit of working out and Parkinson's is not in an advanced stage, then working with a few water weights, gloves, or a noodle should be fine. However if the person is not in the habit of working out and/or the disease is more advanced, than it would be best to use only the water first before adding any equipment. If equipment is used incorrectly, the person could be injured. The purpose of exercise is to maintain and improve the body, not to injure it.

24. Is water exercise financially affordable?

If water exercises are going to become an important part of the participant's life, then it is important to make them affordable. Taking the opportunity to remain as self-sufficient as possible for as long as possible will keep the expense of dependent care at a minimum.

If the person with Parkinson's already belongs to a health club or similar facility, use of the pool is usually included in the membership privileges. If a person is committed to an exercise program, then a health club membership is worth the investment. The person with Parkinson's must weigh financial output and the advantages of an independent lifestyle verses the expense of dependent care and all that kind of care involves.

25. How long can a person live with Parkinson's disease?

Parkinson's disease affects the quality of a person's life rather than life expectancy. Many people live several decades with PD. The leading cause of death among those with PD is respiratory and circulatory complications such as pneumonia and heart disease. People with PD tend to succumb to the same diseases as the general population and at the same age.

The greatest risk factor for people with Parkinson's and not the general population is gait disturbance. The loss of balance contributes to falls and, in an older population, falls can be fatal. Since a person can live a long time with PD, it is wise to focus on maintaining an independent, high quality of life through exercise, diet, and medication.

26. Does Parkinson's disease progress at the same rate with or without medication?

Without drug treatment, Parkinson's would most certainly advance at a faster rate. Unfortunately, Parkinson's disease is a chronic, progressive condition that gets worse over time. The rate of progression varies with different people. Medications for Parkinson's are designed to slow down the rate of neuronal cell death. There have been experimental studies with a drug called Selegiline that suggest it may protect dopamine nerves from degeneration. Other studies are looking at drugs that are designed to stop or slow down the rate of cell death. Letterio Margante published a study in *The Journal of the American Medical Association* on the survival rate of people with Parkinson's. Pneumonia was the most common cause of death. However, a lack of levodopa therapy was cited as a common cause for lower survival rates.

27. Does stress have an effect on the symptoms of Parkinson's disease?

Yes. Momentary stress can temporarily cause symptoms to become worse but momentary stress does not have a permanent effect on Parkinson's disease. For example momentary stress might be worrying about children not coming home from school on time, meeting new in-laws, being stuck in traffic, or missing an appointment. This may cause a person to experience worsening tremors or more severe rigidity. The severity of the symptoms subsides with the removal of the stress.

Long-term, on-going stress can have a permanent effect on Parkinson's symptoms. Long-term stress can lead to depression, which suppresses the immune system, and affects how medication is absorbed. Depression also has an adverse affect on how well a person copes with everyday activities. Exercise is a great stress reliever and boosts the levels of endorphins that alleviate depression.

28. Will I pass Parkinson's disease onto my children?

Parkinson's is not considered a hereditary disease. However, there is a slightly increased incidence of Parkinson's in families where a member has the disease. Families with a history of Parkinson's disease have a 5-10% greater chance of having a family member contract the disease. This may be because family members are exposed to some environmental agent and/or they may share a genetic predisposition to Parkinson's.

28. What are endorphins and how are they affected by exercise?

Endorphins are a class of neurotransmitters that are formed by the body to relieve pain. They are similar to the pain-relieving drug morphine. Endorphins are produced by the pituitary gland and act on certain sites in the brain called opiate receptors that block pain sensations. They also control how the body responds to stress, determine mood, and regulate the contraction of the intestinal wall. Endorphins may also regulate the release of growth hormone. Aerobic exercise and weight training stimulate the release of endorphins, creating a euphoric feeling. This is why exercise generates an overall positive feeling and why exercise is helpful in alleviating depression.

30. Why isn't there a cure for Parkinson's?

There is funding for Parkinson's research but more than money is needed to find a cure. As of now, researchers don't know what the exact cause of PD is or if there is more than one way to get PD.

Although there is research that points to environmental factors and genetic factors for people under 50, more research is needed to find out exactly how it starts. Part of curing a disease is understanding how it starts and progresses. Once that information is known, not only might it be possible to find a cure, it may also be possible to prevent the disease altogether. Researchers, scientists, and physicians are constantly looking for better ways to treat the symptoms of Parkinson's and to slow down its progress.

Recent studies have shown that people who smoke and/or drink coffee have a smaller risk of getting Parkinson's. In one study done at the U.S. Department of Veterans Affairs in Honolulu, 8000 men of Japanese ancestry were admitted into the Honolulu Heart Program. During the 1960's and 1970's, the men's diets were monitored. Over a thirty-year period, 102 of these men developed Parkinson's disease. Of the men studied, those who did not drink coffee or other caffinated beverages on a regular basis had a two to three times greater risk of developing Parkinson's.

Other studies involving nicotine show that when nicotine enters the brain, it stimulates the production of dopamine. Nicotine mimics another neurotransmitter called acetylcholine. Dopamine producing nerve cells have acetylcholine receptor molecules on their surface. Nicotinic receptors have acetylcholine molecules. This scenario causes a cell to produce dopamine. Nicotine is similar enough to acetylcholine to adhere to acetylcholine receptors thus encouraging dopamine production.

Dr. Paul Newhouse, a psychiatrist at the University of Vermont, has been experimenting with nicotine and its effects on people who have Parkinson's. He has noted that people with Parkinson's are able to walk, stand, and resume sitting with more stability after a dose of nicotine. People with Parkinson's also had enhanced learning and memory skills after a dose of nicotine.

Nicotine has many unsafe and undesirable side effects. Drug companies are trying to produce a safe and effective drug that will capture the beneficial qualities of nicotine. Abbott Laboratories has started to test market a compound called ABT-418 that stimulates nicotinic receptors. Dr. Newhouse has tried ABT-418 on a small number of his patients with promising results.

Alcohol consumption also appears to have a relationship to Parkinson's disease. At Stanford University in California, Dr. Loren Nelson has researched the effects of alcohol and how it affects Parkinson's disease. She discovered that regular drinkers, those who consumed 5 to 7 drinks a week, when compared to a control group of non-drinkers, showed a 30% reduction of risk for Parkinson's. Among heavier drinkers, defined as 9 or more drinks a week, the risk reduction was 36%.

The studies mentioned and their results are not meant to advocate or endorse consumption of alcohol, caffeine, and/or nicotine in order to prevent getting Parkinson's disease. These studies do indicate that perhaps some of the chemicals in these products could be extracted and reconstituted into a safe and effective product that may be beneficial in preventing Parkinson's disease. Although the research is interesting and promising, more study is needed.

If a person who has Parkinson's is interested in participating in any clinical trials, here are two addresses of organizations that may be contacted.

National Institute of Neurological Disorders and Stroke (NINDS)
National Institute of Health
9000 Rockville Pike
Bethesda, MD 20892
Tel: (301) 498-6609
Web Site: http://www.nih.gov/science/campus

Parkinson Study Group (PSG)
Clinical Trials Coordination Center
The Mount Hope Professional Building
1351 Mount Hope Avenue
Rochester, NY 14620
Tel: (716) 275-7311
Fax: (716) 461-3554

There are many other organizations that are devoted to finding a cure for PD. Some of the better-known organizations are

American Parkinson Disease Association, Inc.
1250 Hylan Blvd Suite 4B
Staten Island, NY 10305
Tel: (718) 981-8001; (800) 223-2732
Fax: (718) 981-4399
E-mail: info@apdaparkinson.com
Web Site: http://www.apdaparkinson.com

The National Parkinson Foundation, Inc.
1501 NW 9th Ave.
Bob Hope Road
Miami, FL 33136-1494
Tel: (305) 547-6666; (800) 327-4545; in Florida (800) 433-7022
Fax: (305) 243-4403
E-mail: mailbox@npf.med.miami.edu
Web Site: http://www.parkinson.org

Parkinson's Action Network
840 Third Street
Santa Rosa, CA 95405
Tel: (707) 544-1994; (800) 850-4726
Fax: (707) 544-2363
E-mail: info@parkinsonsaction.org
Web Site: www.parkinsonaction.org

The Parkinson's Institute
1170 Morse Ave
Sunnyvale, CA 94089-1605
Tel: (408) 734-2800
E-mail: outreach@parkinsoninstitute.org
Web Site: www.parkinsoninstitute.org

The American Academy of Neurology
1080 Montreal Avenue
St. Paul, MN 55116-2325

Parkinson's Disease Foundation, Inc.
710 West 168th Street
New York, NY 10032-9982
Tel: (212) 923-4700; (800) 457-6676
Fax: (212) 923-4778
E-mail: info@pdf.org
Web Site: www.parkinsons-foundation.org

National Institute of Neurological Disorders and Stroke
PO Box 5801
Bethesda, MD 20824
Tel: (800) 352-9424
E-mail: nindswbadmin@nih.gov
Web Site: www.ninds.nih.gov

The Parkinson Foundation of Canada
390 Bay Street, Suite 710
Toronto, Ontario, Canada M5H 2Y2
Tel: (416) 366-0099; (800) 565-3000 (Canada only)
E-mail: alicia.pace@parkinson.ca
Web Site: www.parkinson.ca

There are many other organizations, and most of the information
about them can be found in the telephone book, the local public
library, or over the Internet.

11. Summary

Exercise is an important part of an overall therapy program for managing Parkinson's disease. Water exercise is ideal for people with Parkinson's. Water exercise helps people living with Parkinson's improve their mobility. Exercising in the water improves balance, strength, and gait problems as well as the emotional well being of people with Parkinson's by giving them a feeling of personal accomplishment. Numerous clinical studies have shown that exercise improves the movements associated with balance and coordination that are affected by Parkinson's disease.

Many physicians strongly recommend an exercise program to help strengthen underused muscles and to put rigid muscles through their full range of motion. Exercise will not cure or stop the progression of Parkinson's disease. It will help to improve body strength and balance so the person with Parkinson's is better able to lead an independent, active life for an extended period of time.

Water exercise provides the person with Parkinson's with the resistance of water, which imitates the action of lifting weights, only it is smoother and more consistent. The muscles are put through a full range of motion and gain strength without causing stress or strain to the joints. Stronger, flexible muscles help the person with Parkinson's improve and maintain an upright gait and improve overall motor function.

As the disease progresses, the person with Parkinson's may want to work with a partner. That partner will have to be aware of the physical abilities, the medications, and their effects. If the person with Parkinson's works out with a partner, his/her partner's role is to support the person with Parkinson's in the pool. His/her partner watches and guides him/her through the exercises correctly using effective visual and verbal cueing. This will help the person with Parkinson's to complete the exercises to his/her full potential.

For safety reasons, the person with Parkinson's should locate a facility that has an easily accessible pool for people with physical disabilities. The goal of water therapy is to keep a person as functional as possible within that person's limitations.

The water's buoyancy allows the person with Parkinson's to perform exercises safely without the risk of injury and strain that can occur in non-water exercises. People with Parkinson's are able to exercise in the water throughout the many stages of their disease because the water's buoyancy helps them control their ability to balance. Use of water equipment helps to supplement the resistance of the water allowing the muscles to work at their full capacity. This equipment can also be used to help stabilize the person with Parkinson's while s/he works in the water.

I have used the techniques described in this book and I know they will improve the lives of people with Parkinson's disease. My sincere hope is that through water exercise, people can enjoy longer, more independent, and more fulfilling lives.

Glossary

abduction: movement away from the midline of the body.

acetylcholine: a chemical messenger that is found in many parts of the body including the brain. Acetylcholine is necessary for normal body functions and has a reciprocal relationship with the brain chemical dopamine. Acetylcholine is involved in the transmission of nerve impulses.

action tremor: an involuntary movement of a limb that is triggered by an initiated movement such as the movement of lifting an object.

adduction: movement towards the midline of the body.

adrenaline: a chemical found in the body; the neurotransmitter that is released by the adrenal gland in a moment of crisis or excitement; also known as epinephrine.

aerobics: a method of exercise such as jogging, swimming, cycling, or any vigorous sustained exercise that is designed to improve circulatory and respiratory efficiency thus improving the body's ability to utilize oxygen.

agonist: a drug or chemical that simulates neurotransmitter activity.

agonist muscle: a muscle that is a prime mover. A specific movement is made by the contraction of the agonist. An example would be the biceps in a bicep curl.

akinesia: impaired muscle movement due to a loss of motor function.

amantadine: a drug that helps the brain release dopamine.

amino acids: strands of any large group of organic compounds comprised of carbon, hydrogen, nitrogen, and oxygen. Amino acids are the basic components of proteins.

anaerobic: exercise requiring more oxygen than the body can take in during the exercise.

Annonaceae: genus of plants whose fruits have neurotoxins that seem to cause atypical Parkinson's in older people.

antagonist muscle: a muscle that is a prime mover and counteracts the movement of the agonist. Agonist and antagonist muscles occur in pairs and are functionally opposite. Such pairs are biceps/triceps, quadriceps/hamstrings.

anterior: in front of the body.

anticholinergic: a type of medication that inhibits the action of acetylcholine. Such medication helps to reduce the tremors, rigidity, and drooling which are associated with Parkinson's.

antihistamines: drugs used to relieve symptoms of colds or allergy, which may also be effective in reducing tremor. Often sold as over-the-counter medications.

antioxidants: nutrients that protect cells and cellular DNA from destruction or mutation.

apomorphine: a dopamine agonist that is derived from morphine and is currently being used as an experimental treatment for severe cases of Parkinson's.

ataxia: inability to coordinate movement and balance.

athetosis: abnormal movements of voluntary muscles that are repetitive and slow.

atrophy: loss of muscle tissue due to lack of use.

atypical: not conforming to a type; unusual.

axial: forming an axis.

axial range of motion: movement originating from an axial point. Examples are movement from the shoulder joint and from the hip joint.

balance: controlling the body's center of gravity to remain in a desired posture.

ballistic stretching: bouncing or tugging a muscle while stretching. Ballistic stretching can cause a muscle to be pulled.

basal ganglia: areas in the brain associated with walking and normal movement.

benzyltetrahydroisoquinoline alkaloids: neurotoxic compounds found in fruits from the plants in the Annonaceae genus. Such fruits include pomme-cannelle, soursop, and custard apple.

beta-blockers: drugs that block the action of epinephrine; usually used to treat heart disease and hypertension.

bilateral: affecting two sides equally.

bradykinesia: a slowing down of movement causing difficulty in executing repetitive movements and fine motor movements.

bradyphrenia: slowness of the thought processes.

buoyancy: the ability to float.

caffeine: a bitter tasting stimulant found in coffee, tea, cola, and some other soft drinks.

carbohydrates: nutrients composed of simple or complex sugars or starches.

cardiovascular disease: disease of the heart and blood vessels.

cardiovascular system: a system made up of the heart and blood vessels in which the blood distributes oxygen and nutrients to the cells of the body and removes carbon dioxide and wastes from the cells.

cascara: herb used to ease the symptoms of constipation.

cayenne: strong red pepper.

chamomile: herb often used in tea form to counter the effects of indigestion.

chaparral: herb that is touted as a cancer cure but has very serious side effects and lacks scientific proof.

chlorine: chemical used to disinfect water; commonly used in swimming pools.

cholesterol: white crystalline substance found in animal tissue and other foods. Cholesterol is important to the development of cell membranes but too much of the wrong kind can cause heath problems.

choline: a precursor of acetylcholine.

chorea: a type of abnormal movement that is continuous, rapid, and dance-like. This kind of dyskinesia may result from high doses of levodopa, although it has many other causes. Long-term use of levodopa can also result in chorea.

choreoathetosis: a type of dyskinesia that is characterized by both chorea and athetosis movements.

cogwheel rigidity: a stiffness of the muscles that causes movement to be jerky and uneven.

comfrey: common herb that some claim has the ability to purify the blood. It has serious side effects.

cortisol: stress-depression hormone.

CPR: cardiopulmonary resuscitation.

custard apple: Tropical heart-shaped fruit with white or yellowish flesh.

dementia: a progressive mental condition manifested by increasing confusion, disorientation, and disintegration of the personality.

depreny: a drug such as Eldepryl, Selegiline, and Jumex that increases the effects of dopamine in the brain.

disequilibrium: loss of balance.

dopa decarboxylase inhibitors: drugs which block levodopa's conversion to dopamine outside of the brain.

dopamine: a chemical produced by the brain that controls the actions of movement, balance, and walking.

dopamine agonist: drugs that imitate the effects of dopamine.

drag: the resistance force that acts on an object moving through liquid or air.

drug holiday: withdrawal of a drug after long-term treatment.

drug induced: brought about through drug use.

dry ramp: method of pool entry.

duration: the amount of time spent.

dysarthria: difficulty coordinating or using the muscles associated with speech.

dyskinesia: the abnormal movement of voluntary muscles. Athetosis, chorea, and dystonia are all types of dyskinesia.

dysphagia: swallowing difficulty.

dystonia: slow movement or prolonged spasm in a muscle group; most often affects the head, neck, and tongue.

edema: abnormal accumulation of fluid; leads to swelling of the limbs.

endorphins: class of neurotransmitters produced by the pituitary gland that controls the sensation of pain and gives a person an overall positive feeling. Exercise is one activity that stimulates the release of endorphins.

ephedra: herb used to induce weight loss. It is a strong stimulant with serious side effects.

extension: bending backwards or straightening out.

fats: oily, solid material found in animal tissue.

festination: a way of walking using short, shuffling steps.

flexibility: the ability of a muscle or joint to stretch and move freely.

flexion: bending forwards or decreasing the angle of a joint.

flotation device: equipment used in the water that floats. It is used to add more resistance during water exercise and to help a person maintain stability. Some flotation devices can help a person float but not all.

freezing: an involuntary, temporary inability to move.

frequency: how often a person performs an exercise (or some other action).

frontal plane: imaginary plane that divides the body into front and back halves.

ginger: herb used to help suppress nausea.

ginkgo biloba: herb used for many cognitive changes; has some side effects.

glaucoma: impaired vision or blindness due to an injured optic nerve caused by high pressure inside the eye. Anticholinergics may exacerbate the condition.

HDL: high-density lipids; the "good" cholesterol.

heterogeneous: having dissimilar qualities; unlike.

Hoehn and Yahr Stages: common rating scale used to measure the progression of Parkinson's disease. The stages are

1. Unilateral involvement with minimal or no functional impairment.
2. Bilateral involvement or midline involvement without impairment of balance.

3. First sign of impaired righting reflexes evident by unsteadiness as the patient turns or is pushed from standing equilibrium with feet together and eyes closed.
4. Fully developed, person is severely disabled, but is still able to walk and stand without assistance although is markedly incapacitated.
5. Confined to bed or wheelchair, no movement unless assisted.

Huperzine A: Chinese herb that is supposed to help restore acetylcholine.

hydrocarbon: any organic compound that contains only carbon and hydrogen.

hydrostatic pressure: pressure from liquid upon an immersed object.

hypokinesia: motor activity that is abnormally diminished.

idiopathic: from an unknown cause. The most common form of Parkinson's disease is idiopathic.

intensity: the amount of energy expended during exercise.

intention tremor: a tremor that occurs when a person executes a voluntary movement.

kickboards: buoyant, durable, lightweight flat boards that can be used to help a person support himself/herself in the water while performing exercises.

kyphosis: exaggerated curvature of the upper spine. The head is too far forwards and the shoulders appear rounded.

lateral: towards the side; away from the midline.

LDL: low density lipids; the "bad" cholesterol.

levodopa: a generic name for L-Dopa; contained in the drugs Sinemet and Atamet.

levodopa-induced dyskinesia: abnormal, involuntary movements that are a side effect of prolonged levodopa use. Reducing the amount of levodopa may alleviate levodopa-induced dyskinesia.

lift: chair or sling used to bring a person from the edge of a pool into the pool.

livedo reticularis: a benign skin condition that is found in some people taking the drug amantadine marketed under the name Symmetrel. The condition causes purplish or bluish mottling of the skin below the knee and sometimes on the forearms.

lobelia: herb that supposedly enhances respiratory function. Also known as pukeweed and can be toxic.

maneb: a fungicide that is widely used and may be linked to Parkinson's

maximum heart rate: the fastest rate at which the heart beats during aerobic activity. To calculate MHR: take 220 and subtract your age if male; take 226 and subtract your age if female. It is assumed that females have smaller hearts that beat faster to do the same amount of work. Therefore, males use 220 as a base number and females use 226. Some drugs have significant effects on the ability of the heart to change rate. If there are any questions, ask your physician before strenuous exercise.

medial: towards the midline dividing the body into left and right sides.

micrographia: small, cramped handwriting due to decreased ability to utilize fine motor movements as a result of Parkinson's.

minerals: naturally occurring inorganic substances.

moveable floors: method of pool entry.

MPTP: a toxic chemical. Some researchers believe that exposure to this can lead to Parkinson's disease.

myoclonus: involuntary, jerky movement of extremities during sleep.

neuroleptic drugs: drugs that act as dopamine antagonists.

neurotransmitter: a chemical produced in nerve cells that transmits information between nerve cells.

nicotine: oily liquid that comes from the tobacco plant.

nigrostriatal degeneration: degeneration caused by dopamine that damages the pathways that are affected by Parkinson's between the substantia nigra and the striatum of the brain.

norepinephrine: a chemical transmitter in the brain that governs the involuntary autonomic nervous system.

on-off phenomenon: the fluctuation between a good response (on) and a poor response (off) that occurs suddenly and unpredictably. This on-off phenomenon is found in people who are on levodopa therapy.

orthostatic hypotension: a drop in blood pressure brought on by a sudden change in body position. An example would be a lighted-headed feeling one might get from standing up out of a chair too quickly.

over gripping: holding an object with too much force; squeezing.

palilalia: interrupted speech flow when the person with Parkinson's repeats a word or syllable.

paralysis agitans: the Latin term that means shaking palsy; the phrase used to describe Parkinson's disease before James Parkinson's time.

paraquat: a herbicide that is widely used and may be linked to Parkinson's.

paresthesia: the spontaneous sensation of "pins and needles" felt in an extremity or other part of the body.

Parkinsonism: a clinical state where a person exhibits classic

Parkinson symptoms such as a tremor, rigidity, stooped posture, and bradykinesia. The cause for Parkinsonism is still unknown. Reversible Parkinsonism can be drug induced.

Parkinson's disease: the form of Parkinsonism named by James Parkinson. He described the disease as a chronic, progressive disease that affects the nervous system. Symptoms include tremor, rigidity, bradykinesia, and a stooped posture.

Parkinson's facies: a mask-like, emotionless expression of the face with infrequent blinking of the eyes.

Parlodel: a dopamine agonist used to treat Parkinson's primary symptoms.

peppermint: herb used in tea form to offset symptoms of indigestion.

Permax: a dopamine agonist, stronger than Parlodel.

pomme cannelle: fruit from the Annonacea genus that contains neurotoxins shown to cause atypical Parkinson's in the elderly.

posterior: the back of the body or body part.

postural deformity: stooped posture.

postural instability: inability to balance caused by postural problems.

postural tremor: tremor that increases in severity when the hands are stretched out in front. Also known as sustention tremor.

Prolopa: An antiparkinson drug made of 4 mg levodopa to 1 mg of benserazide.

prone: lying face down.

propulsive gait: much like festination but the steps progress from walking to running in shorter and faster steps and may cause falling.

range of motion (ROM): the distance that a joint is able to move between fully straight to completely bent.

receptor: a sensory nerve that reacts to stimulus.

resting tremor: shaking of a relaxed and supported limb.

retropulsive gait: backwards propulsive gait.

rigidity: muscular stiffness that is resistant to passive manipulation.

St. John's wort: herb used to relieve mild symptoms of depression.

saw palmetto: herb used by men to help with symptoms of urinary problems.

Schwab and England Activities of Daily Living Assessment: an assessment of people with Parkinson's that looks at how dependent they are in performing activities of daily living

senna: herb used to help alleviate symptoms of constipation.

sialorrhea: drooling.

side effect: an effect produced by a drug that is in addition to its beneficial effects; usually undesirable.

Sinemet: an antiparkinson drug that is either 4 mg or 10 mg of levodopa to 1 mg of carbidopa.

Sinemet CR: the same drug as Sinemet but in a controlled released capsule allowing the drug to be released into the body more slowly.

soursop: tropical evergreen tree that bears a tart spiny fruit from the Annonacea genus. The fruit contains neurotoxins that cause atypical Parkinson's in the elderly.

spasm: involuntary contraction of a muscle or group of muscles.

stretching: a specific type of exercise that increases the ability of a joint or muscle to reach, bend, or turn.

striatum: the area of the brain responsible for controlling walking, balance, and movement. The striatum connects to and receives transmissions from the substantia nigra.

substantia nigra: area of the brain where dopamine is made.

supine: lying face up.

sustention tremor: See postural tremor.

Symmetrel: market name for the drug Amantadine.

target heart rate (THR): a percentage of the maximum heart rate (MHR) achieved during exercise. THR can be between 60-90% of the MHR depending on the fitness level of the individual.

toxin: poisonous substance.

tremor: sequential muscle contractions that cause rhythmic, involuntary shaking of the body or body parts.

unilateral: affecting one side of the body. The symptoms of Parkinson's start unilaterally.

United Parkinson's Disease Rating Scale (UPDRS): an in depth evaluation of the mental abilities, behavior, mood, level of daily activities, and motor skills of people with Parkinson's

valerian root: herb used to offset sleep and anxiety problems. Has side effects.

vomiting center: area of the brain controlling nausea and vomiting. May be affected by some medications.

wearing-off phenomenon: refers to the waning effects of the last dose of levodopa.

yohimbine: herb marketed as a muscle enhancer, body fat reducer, and aphrodisiac. Has serious side effects.

zero-depth entry: gentle sloping ramp into a pool.

Bibliography

3 Win for Work on Brain Cells' Function: Insights Gained on Memory, Neurological Disorders. (2000, October 10). *Startribune*, Metro ed. Minneapolis, MN. p. 01A.

Ahrens, T. (1999). Exercise to Your Heart's Content. *Current Health, 25*(15):13.

American College of Physicians. (2000). *Home Medical Guide to Parkinson's Disease.* New York, NY: Dorling Kindersley Book.

Argue, J. (2000). *Parkinson's Disease & the Art of Moving.* Oakland, CA: New Harbinger Publications, Inc.

Austin, R. (1994). *Relationship Between Stage and Strength for People with Parkinson's Disease.* Ann Arbor, MN: U.M.I. Dissertation Services.

AWE-some: Adult Wellness Exercise Program. (1992) Video. Staten Island, NY: The American Parkinson Disease Association.

Biziere, K. & Kurth, M. (1997). *Living with Parkinson's Disease.* New York, NY: Demos Vermande.

Bridges, B. (1995). *Therapeutic Caregiving: A Practical Guide for Caregivers of Persons with Alzheimer's and Other Dementia Causing Diseases.* Mill Creek, WA: BJB Publishing.

Bridgewater, K. & Sharpe, M. (1998). Trunk Muscle Performance in Early Parkinson's Disease. *Physical Therapy 78*(6):566-76.

Broach, E. & Datillo, J. (1996). Aquatic Therapy: Making Waves in Therapeutic Recreation. *Parks and Recreation 31*(7):38-42.

Bruman, J. (2000). *Secondary Symptoms of PD.* http://www.geocities.com/janet313/pienet/bruman/index.html

Carter, J. (1992). *Good Nutrition in Parkinson's Disease.* Staten Island, NY: American Parkinson Disease Association, Inc.

Case, L. (1997). *Fitness Aquatics.* Champaign, IL: Human Kinetics.

Childers, C. (2000). Therapeutic Value of Exercise Training in Parkinson's Disease. *Physical Therapy 80*(5):538.

Clarke, P. (1992) *A Case Study on the Roll of Exercise in the Management of Parkinson's Disease.* Newfoundland: University of Newfoundland.

Coffee May Protect Against Parkinson's Disease. (2000, June 17) *Chemist & Druggist.* p. VI.

Colais-Germain, B. (1993). *Anatomy of Movement.* Seattle, WA: Eastland Press.

Coleman, E. (2000). *Herbs for Health.* www.hcrc.org/coleman/herbs.html

Cote, L. & Riede, G. (1999). *Exercises for the Parkinson's Patient with Hints for Daily Living.* New York, NY: Parkinson's Disease Foundation.

Dorros, S. & Dorros, D. (1992). *Patient Perspectives on Parkinson's; A Series of Essays.* Miami, FL: National Parkinson's Foundation.

Duffy, M. (2000, October). Herbal Enemy No. 1. *Reader's Digest,* p.130.

Duvoisin, J. (1996). *Parkinson's Disease: A Guide for Patient and Family.* Philadelphia, PA: Lippincott-Raven.

Exercise; A Guide from the National Institute on Aging. (1998). National Institutes of Health. Publication No. NIH 99-4258.

Gabrielse, A. (Ed.) (1987). *Swimming Pools: A Guide to Their Planning, Design, and Operation, 4th ed.* Champaign, IL: Human Kinetics, Inc.

Gaines, M. (1993). *Fantastic Water Workouts.* Champaign, IL: Human Kinetics, Inc.

Gardner, J. (2000, Summer). Care Needed in Using Herbs for Parkinson's. *Satellite: A Publication of the Struthers Parkinson's Center Mpls.* p. 1, 3-4.

Gladwin, L (1999). Parkinson's Disease and Exercise. *American Fitness. 17*(3):51-55.

Great Drug, Shame about the Delivery System. (Health Aspects of Tobacco) (2000, September 23). *The Economist (U.S.), 356* (8189):95.

Gringsby, L. (1993). *Aquatic Therapy Helps.* www.webco.net/apda/physical/aqua.htm

Hauser, R. & Zesiewicz, T. (1997). *Parkinson's Disease: Questions and Answers.* Coral Springs, Fl: Merit Publications International.

Head, E. (1997). Balance Activities in Parkinson's Disease. Somerset Pharmaceuticals, Inc. Mylan Laboratories Inc. www.somersetpharm.com

Henderson, C. (2001, January 27). Combination of two widely used pesticides linked to disease. (Paraquat and Maneb linked to Parkinson's disease). *Pain & Central Nervous System Week,* p. 9.

Hirsch, M., Rider, R., Toole, T., & Hirsch, H. (1998). Developing a Balance and Resistance Training Program (Falls Prevention in Individuals with Parkinson' Disease, part 2). *Palaestra 14*(14):21.

Hirsch, M., Rider, R., Toole, T. & Hirsch, H. (1998). Falls Prevention in Individuals with Parkinson's Disease. *Palaestra 14*(3):15-20.

Huey, L. & Robert F. (1993). *The Complete Waterpower Workout Book.* New York, NY: Random House.

Hussar, D. (1999). New Drugs 99. *Nursing 29*(2):45.

Hutton, T. & Dippel, R. (1989). *Caring for the Parkinson Patient: A Practical Guide.* Buffalo, New York: Prometheus Books.

In Brief; Coffee in Moderation Linked to Lower Parkinson's Risk. (2000, October 25). *Startribune* Metro ed. Minneapolis, MN p. 05E.

Jahanshahi, M. & Marsden, C. (2000). *Parkinson's Disease: A Self-help Guide.* New York, NY: Demos Medical Publishing, Inc.

Jeffery, S. (1999). Patient's Bad Habits Make Parkinson's Less of a Threat. *Medical Post. 35*(23). www.medicalpost.com/mdlink.

J. M. (2000). Exercise Eases Parkinson's (Studies in Germany Indicate Beneficial Results from Exercise for Parkinson's Disease Victims). *Prevention 5*(6):174.

Johnson, A. (Ed.). (1995). *Young Parkinson's Handbook.* Staten Island, New York: The American Parkinson Disease Association.

Johnston, M. (2000). Water Exercise for Parkinson's Disease and Other Movement Disorders. Body Check Inc. www.waterart.org/newsletter13.htm

Katz, J. (1985). *The W.E.T. Workout: Water Exercises Techniques to Help You Tone Up and Slim Down Aerobically.* New York: Facts on File Publications.

Kennedy, C. (1997). Aquatic Fitness: Making the Water Work for You. *Parks and Recreation 32*(2):48-52.

Klosterman, K. (1995). *Parkinson's Disease: An Exercise Approach to Treatment.* Dissertation, University of North Dakota, Grand Forks, ND.

Lieberman, A. (1993). *Parkinson's Disease: The Complete Guide for Patients and Caregivers.* New York, NY: Simon and Schuster.

Lieberman, A., Gopinathan, G., Neophytide, A. & Goldstein, M. (1995). *Parkinson's Disease Handbook.* Staten Island, New York: The American Parkinson Disease Association.

Lieberman, A. (2001). *Does Where You Live Matter?* National Parkinson Foundation. http://www.parkinson.org/surveys.htm

Liebman, B. (2000). Caffeine & Parkinson's Disease. *Nutrition Action Health Letter 27*(7):11.

Lindle, J. (Ed.). (1995). *Aquatic Fitness Professional Manual.* Nokomis, FL: Aquatic Exercise Association.

Macmillan Health Encyclopedia. (1993). *Vol. 1 Body and Systems.* New York, NY: Macmillan Publishing Company.

Matus, J. (2000). Nicotine Remedy for Alzheimer's and Parkinson's. *Prevention 52*(8):171.

Millard, T. (1992). *The Effect of Cardiovascular Training on Fitness and Motor Performance in Parkinson's Disease.* Emory University School of Medicine.

Mitchell, E. & Rutheford, M. (1998, November 30). Life Stretches: Yoga, QiGong, Pilate's and a New Wave of Water Exercises are Fast Becoming the Post 50 Generation's Choice Workouts. *Time Magazine.* p. 128.

Molkentin, S. (1997). *Depression and Parkinson's Disease.* Somerset Pharmaceuticals, Inc. Mylan Laboratories Inc.

Morgante, L. (2000). Parkinson's Disease Survival: A Population-Based Study. *Journal of the American Medical Association 284*(6):676.

Mraz, Tom. Written letter. April 1999.

Organic Solvents Increase Parkinson's Risk (September 18, 2000). *Chemistry and Industry,* p. 59.

Osinski, A. (1998). ADA Compliance for Pools and Wet Access. *Fitness Management Magazine 14*(5).

Paciorek, M. & Jones, J. (1989). *Sports and Recreation for the Disabled: A Resource Manual.* Indianapolis, IN: Benchmark Press Inc.

Parkinson's Disease Handbook, A Guide for Patients and Their Families. (1998). Staten Island New York: The American Parkinson Disease Association.

Parkinson's Disease: Hope Through Research. (1994 September). Bethesda, MD: National Institute of Neurological Disorders and Stroke.

Parkinson's Disease Medication: Tasmar. (1998). Clinical Tools, Inc.

Pesticide Rotenone Found to Produce Parkinson's Disease Symptoms in Rats. (2000, November 5). *Startribune*, Metro ed., Minneapolis, MN. p. A11.

Phillips, P. (1999a, September 8). Several Classes of New Drugs Emerging for Parkinson Disease. *The Journal of the American Medical Association 282*(10):929.

Phillips, P. (1999b). Keeping Depression at Bay Helps Patients with Parkinson Disease. *The Journal of the American Medical Association. 282(*12):1118.

Posner, C. & Ronthal, M. (1991, December). Exercise and Alzheimer's Disease, Parkinson's Disease, and Multiple Sclerosis. *The Physician and Sports Medicine 19*(12):85-92.

Schenman, M., Outson, T., Kuchibnatla, M., Chandler, J., Pieper, C., Ray, L. & Laub, K. (1998). Exercise to Improve Spinal Flexibility and Function for People with PD: A Randomized Controlled Trial. *Journal of the American Geriatrics Society 46*(10):1207-1217.

Seppa, N. (1999). Tropical Fruits Linked to Parkinsonism. (Indications that the Three Tropical Fruits Soursop, Custard Apple, and Pomme Cannelle May Result in Parkinson's-like Illnesses). *Science News 156*(5):69.

Smith, Ann. *Water Therapy.* APDA Great Plains Parkinson Corporation. October, 1999, www.webco.net/apda/physical/water.

Sobel, R. (2000, June 5). A Cappuccino a Day. *U.S. News & World Report 128*(22):63.

Stanley, Rhonda K. (1996). *Exercise Intervention in Males and Females Having Idiopathic Parkinson's Disease.* Dissertation Texas Woman's University School of Physical Therapy. Houston, Texas.

Wachmann, R. (1990). *Be Active: A Suggested Exercise Program for People with Parkinson's Disease.* Minneapolis, MN: APDA The Institute for Rehabilitation Services, Methodist Hospital.

Water Exercise Fact Sheet. www.vtc.vsc.edu/shape/programs/wfact.html

Water Exercises for Parkinson's Disease Patients. (1992). Video. Staten Island, New York: The American Parkinson Disease Association.

Water Sports for the Disabled. (1983). West Yorkshire, England: EP Publishing Ltd.

Watkins, B. & Loverock, P. (1988). *The Water Workout Recovery Program: Safe and Painless Exercises for Treating Back Pain, Muscle Tears, Tendonitis, Sports Injuries and More.* Chicago, IL: Contemporary Books.

Weiner, W. S. & Lang, A. L. (2001). *Parkinson's Disease; A Complete Guide For Patients and Families*. Baltimore, MD: John Hopkins University Press.

Wichman, R., Walde-Douglas, M & Harris, C. (1998). *Parkinson's Disease: Fitness Counts*. Miami, FL: National Parkinson's Foundation Inc.

Wylle, Mary. (1997). *Texas Health Resources*. Fogelson Center for Parkinson's Disease and Neurological Disorders.
http://159.65.68.201/clinsvcs/senrmeds.htm

Index

About the Author

Ann Rosenstein has been teaching water aerobics and other fitness classes since 1989. She is certified through the Aerobics and Fitness Association of America (AFAA), the Aquatic Education Association, Mad Dog (indoor cycling), and the Physicalmind Institute. Ms. Rosenstein instructs water aerobics, indoor cycling, indoor rowing, weight training, and pilates for the Northwest Athletic Club. She is also a certified personal trainer (AFAA) and was named instructor of the year by the Northwest Athletic Club in 1999.

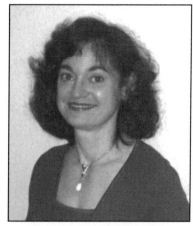

Ann has a B.A. and an M.A. degree from the University of Minnesota. She is employed as a reference librarian as well as a fitness instructor. Her hobbies include Tae Kwon Do, jogging, and music.

She makes her home in Burnsville, Minnesota where she lives with her husband, Leo, daughter, Sarah, and son, Ben.